The Complete

RENAL DIET
COOKBOOK

—— for Beginners ——

The Complete Renal Diet Cookbook for Beginners:
Kidney Disease Management with Simple & Delicious Kidney-Friendly Recipes
for Over 2700 Days — Includes 12–Week Meal Plan & Nutritional Guide

Jessica C. Harper

Copyright Notice

Disclaimer

Contents

———

CHAPTER 8

Snacks & Side Dishes........................ 81

CHAPTER 9

Desserts 98

CHAPTER 10

Beverages 111

CHAPTER 11

CHAPTER 12 (BONUS CHAPTER)

CHAPTER 1

Introduction to Kidney Health and Renal Diet

———

Welcome to "The Complete Renal Diet Cookbook for Beginners. It is not just a book;
it's a new beginning, a guide crafted with care, dedication, and a deep understanding of
the challenges those navigating kidney health issues face.

This book's heart lies in a simple yet profound premise: What we eat significantly impacts our kidney health and overall well-being. Whether you are newly diagnosed with kidney disease, seeking to prevent kidney issues, or caring for someone who is, this book is your companion. It is designed to demystify the renal diet, making it accessible, manageable, and, most importantly, enjoyable.

But this book offers more than just recipes. It serves as an educational tool, providing readers with a solid understanding of kidney function, the impact of diet on kidney health, and practical advice on navigating everyday challenges. You'll learn about the essential nutrients to monitor, how to read food labels effectively, and tips for meal planning and grocery shopping.

AFTER READING THIS BOOK, YOU WILL GAIN:

- A deeper understanding of how diet influences kidney function and overall health.
- Practical skills to prepare delicious, kidney-friendly meals without compromising on taste.
- Strategies to adapt your diet to fit your lifestyle, making it sustainable and enjoyable.
- Insights into managing dietary challenges during social events, holidays, and dining out ensure you can maintain your renal diet without feeling isolated or restricted.

I invite you to dive into "The Complete Renal Diet Cookbook for Beginners" with an open mind and a willing heart. Let this book guide you in discovering how satisfying and flavorful a renal diet can be. Whether you're taking your first steps toward kidney health or looking to expand your culinary repertoire, this book promises to be a valuable resource, offering encouragement, support, and inspiration every step of the way.

Embrace this opportunity to transform your health, one delicious meal at a time. Welcome to your new beginning.

Understanding Kidney Function

In this subchapter of the "Renal Diet Cookbook for Beginners," we delve into
the fundamental aspects of kidney function, providing a foundational understanding crucial
for appreciating the importance of a renal diet.

THE ROLE OF KIDNEYS IN THE BODY

The kidneys are vital organs with multiple crucial functions. Their primary role is freeing the body from metabolic products and, first of all, nitrogenous products of protein metabolism. This purification process is essential for maintaining a balanced internal environment, which includes regulating the body's fluid levels, electrolyte balance, and acid-base balance.

HOW KIDNEYS WORK

Each kidney contains about a million tiny filtering units called nephrons. Blood enters the kidney, and these nephrons filter out waste products, excess salt, and fluids to form urine. This urine then travels to the bladder and is excreted from the body. Notably, kidneys reabsorb what the body needs while removing waste, such as glucose, amino acids, and water.

REGULATION OF BLOOD PRESSURE AND FLUID BALANCE

Besides waste removal, kidneys play a pivotal role in regulating blood pressure. They do this by controlling the volume of blood (through fluid balance) and the amount of sodium and other electrolytes in the blood. Kidneys release hormones that regulate these functions. For instance, when blood pressure drops, kidneys release renin, a hormone that helps restore blood pressure.

ROLE IN RED BLOOD CELL PRODUCTION AND BONE HEALTH

Kidneys also influence other aspects of health. They produce erythropoietin, a hormone that stimulates the bone marrow to produce red blood cells. Furthermore, they convert vitamin D into an active form, essential for maintaining bone health.

IMPACT OF DIET ON KIDNEY FUNCTION

What you eat significantly impacts your kidney health. A diet high in certain substances, like sodium and phosphorus, can strain the kidneys, mainly if an underlying kidney condition exists. Understanding the intricate work of the kidneys underscores the importance of a renal diet in maintaining kidney health and preventing further damage.

CONCLUSION

One can better appreciate the importance of dietary choices in supporting kidney health by grasping the complexities of how kidneys function and their crucial role in overall health. This knowledge sets the foundation for the subsequent sections, where specific nutritional guidelines and lifestyle adjustments for kidney health are discussed in detail.

Essentials of a Renal Diet

This subchapter focuses on the core principles of a renal diet, which is vital for anyone looking to maintain or improve kidney health. The renal diet is tailored to lessen the kidneys' workload, ensuring they function more efficiently, especially for those with kidney concerns.

PURPOSE OF A RENAL DIET

The primary goal of a renal diet is to decrease the accumulation of certain substances in the blood that kidneys typically filter out. This diet is specifically designed to reduce the strain on kidneys by limiting certain nutrients that can be harmful in excessive amounts for those with compromised kidney function.

KEY NUTRIENTS TO MONITOR

- **Sodium:** Excess sodium can lead to fluid retention and increased blood pressure, taxing the kidneys. A renal diet involves consuming low-sodium foods and avoiding high-salt items.
- **Potassium:** While potassium is essential for nerve and muscle function, impaired kidneys may not filter it effectively. This could lead to dangerously high levels in the blood. The renal diet often involves managing potassium intake.
- **Phosphorus:** High phosphorus levels can cause bone and heart issues in people with kidney disease. Limiting foods high in phosphorus is a critical aspect of the renal diet.
- **Protein:** Although essential, excessive protein can increase kidney workload. The renal diet may involve moderating protein intake, focusing on high-quality sources.

FLUID INTAKE

Depending on individual kidney function, fluid intake may need to be monitored. While adequate hydration is essential, too much fluid can lead to complications in individuals with advanced kidney disease.

BALANCED AND VARIED DIET

While focusing on these restrictions, it's also essential to maintain a balanced diet. This includes consuming various fruits, vegetables, whole grains, and lean proteins tailored to individual nutritional needs and kidney health status.

ADAPTING TO INDIVIDUAL NEEDS

The renal diet isn't one-size-fits-all. It must be adjusted based on the kidney disease stage, other medical conditions, and overall health goals. Consulting with healthcare professionals, including a dietitian, is crucial for tailoring the diet to individual needs.

CONCLUSION

Understanding the essentials of a renal diet is a fundamental step in managing kidney health. It involves knowing what foods to limit or avoid and maintaining a balanced and nutritious diet suited to individual health requirements. The following chapters will delve deeper into specific nutritional guidelines, meal planning, and lifestyle adjustments to align with the principles of a renal diet.

CHAPTER 2

Foods to Include and Avoid

—

In this subchapter of the "Renal Diet Cookbook for Beginners," we will explore specific foods beneficial for kidney health and those that should be limited or avoided in a renal diet. This guidance helps in making informed dietary choices that support kidney function.

FOODS TO INCLUDE

✓ **Low-Potassium Fruits and Vegetables:** Apples, berries, grapes, pineapple, plums, bell peppers, carrots, cauliflower, green beans, lettuce, and onions are good choices. These provide essential nutrients without overloading potassium.

✓ **Lean Proteins:** Incorporate lean meats like chicken, fish, and turkey. Egg whites are also a good source of protein with minimal phosphorus.

✓ **Whole Grains:** Whole grains such as barley, buckwheat, bulgur, and couscous are preferable over refined grains as they provide more fiber and nutrients.

✓ **Heart-Healthy Fats:** Include sources of healthy fats like olive oil, avocado, and unsalted nuts in moderation.

FOODS TO AVOID OR LIMIT

× **High-Sodium Foods:** Processed foods, canned soups, packaged snacks, and deli meats often contain high sodium. Opt for fresh or frozen items and use herbs and spices for flavoring instead of salt.

× **High-Potassium Foods:** Limit or avoid bananas, oranges, potatoes, tomatoes, and spinach, as these are high in potassium.

× **Phosphorus-Rich Foods:** Avoid or limit dairy products, nuts, seeds, beans, and whole grains high in phosphorus. Opt for their lower phosphorus alternatives.

× **Processed and Fast Foods:** These often contain high levels of sodium, phosphorus, and unhealthy fats.

FLUID INTAKE

While not a food, it's essential to discuss fluid intake. Depending on the stage of kidney disease, fluid restrictions may be necessary. Consult with healthcare providers for personalized advice.

ADAPTING TO TASTE PREFERENCES

While following these guidelines, catering to personal taste preferences and cultural dietary habits is essential. Finding a balance between being kidney-friendly and enjoyable is critical to maintaining a sustainable and healthy diet.

CONCLUSION

Identifying foods to include and avoid is critical to managing a renal diet. This chapter provides clear guidelines for making kidney-friendly food choices while ensuring the diet is varied and enjoyable. The following chapters will build on this foundation, offering practical tips for meal planning, grocery shopping, and adapting to lifestyle changes while adhering to these dietary guidelines.

Managing Fluid Intake

UNDERSTANDING THE IMPORTANCE OF FLUID BALANCE

The kidneys play a crucial role in regulating the body's fluid balance. For those with kidney disease, maintaining the right balance of fluids can be challenging. Too much fluid can lead to high blood pressure, swelling, and heart problems, while too little can lead to dehydration.

INDIVIDUALIZED FLUID NEEDS

Fluid needs vary depending on the stage of kidney disease and other health factors. Generally, average fluid intake may not need to be altered in the early stages of kidney disease. However, fluid restrictions may become necessary as kidney function declines, especially in advanced stages.

TIPS FOR MANAGING FLUID INTAKE

- **Measure and Monitor:** Monitor how much fluid is consumed throughout the day. This includes drinks and foods with high water content, like soups, fruits, and vegetables.
- **Control Thirst:** Sipping water throughout the day rather than drinking large amounts at once can help manage thirst. Chewing gum or sucking on hard candy (preferably sugar-free) can also help.
- **Be Aware of Hidden Fluids:** Certain foods, like gelatin, ice cream, and yogurt, contribute to fluid intake.
- **Limit Salt Intake:** Reducing salt consumption can help control thirst and fluid retention.
- **Use Smaller Cups:** Using smaller glasses or cups can help prevent the amount of liquid consumed at one time.
- **Monitor Weight Daily:** Sudden weight gain may indicate fluid retention, signaling a need to adjust fluid intake.

ADJUSTING TO FLUID RESTRICTIONS

Adapting to fluid restrictions can be challenging. It's essential to find strategies that work for individual preferences and lifestyles. Creativity in managing thirst and fluid intake without feeling deprived is critical.

WORKING WITH HEALTHCARE PROFESSIONALS

It's crucial to consult with healthcare professionals to determine personalized fluid intake recommendations. They can provide guidance based on health status, kidney function, and lifestyle factors.

CONCLUSION

Managing fluid intake is a vital component of a renal diet. This chapter provides practical advice on monitoring and controlling fluid consumption, which is essential for individuals with varying stages of kidney disease. Understanding and implementing these strategies will aid in maintaining the delicate balance required for optimal kidney health.

Understanding and Balancing Electrolytes: Sodium, Potassium, and Phosphorus

Managing the balance of electrolytes is crucial for those with kidney concerns, as they play a vital role in overall health and kidney function.

THE ROLE OF ELECTROLYTES IN THE BODY

Electrolytes are minerals in your blood and other body fluids that carry an electric charge. They are essential for many bodily functions, including maintaining fluid balance, muscle contractions, and nerve signaling.

● SODIUM

✓ **Importance:** Sodium helps control blood pressure and regulates fluid balance. However, when kidneys are not functioning optimally, sodium can accumulate, leading to fluid retention and hypertension.

✓ **Management:** A renal diet typically involves limiting sodium intake to prevent these complications. This means avoiding table salt, reducing consumption of high-sodium foods like processed meats, canned soups, and salty snacks, and choosing fresh or frozen foods over processed ones.

▲ POTASSIUM

✓ **Importance:** Potassium is critical for nerve function, muscle control, and heart health. However, impaired kidneys may struggle to maintain proper potassium levels, potentially leading to dangerous heart rhythms.

✓ **Management:** Balancing potassium involves limiting or ensuring adequate intake, depending on kidney function. This might include moderating high-potassium foods like bananas, oranges, potatoes, and tomatoes or providing sufficient intake if levels are low.

■ PHOSPHORUS

✓ **Importance:** Phosphorus is key in bone health, energy production, and cell repair. However, excess phosphorus can be harmful when kidney function is compromised, leading to bone and cardiovascular problems.

✓ **Management:** Managing phosphorus intake typically involves limiting phosphorus-rich foods, such as dairy products, nuts, seeds, beans, and whole grains. The body more readily absorbs phosphorus from animal sources than from plants, so attention to food sources is critical.

BALANCING THROUGH DIET

Managing these electrolytes involves more than just eliminating certain foods. It includes making informed choices about what to eat, how much, and how often. Understanding food labels, portion sizes, and the nutritional content of foods is crucial.

CONSULTATION WITH HEALTHCARE PROFESSIONALS

Given the complexities of electrolyte management in kidney disease, it is essential to work with healthcare professionals. Dietitians can provide tailored advice and meal plans that balance these electrolytes according to individual health needs and kidney function.

CHAPTER 3

Organizing a Kidney-Friendly Kitchen

Setting up your kitchen correctly is crucial in successfully managing a renal diet.
It involves stocking the right foods, using appropriate cooking tools, and organizing the space
to encourage healthy eating habits.

STOCKING THE RIGHT FOODS

- **Pantry Essentials:** Fill your pantry with low-sodium seasonings, herbs, and spices to add flavor without adding salt—stock on kidney-friendly staples like rice, pasta, and low-potassium canned vegetables. Include whole grains and beans (if appropriate for your stage of kidney disease).

- **Refrigerator and Freezer:** Keep fresh and frozen fruits and vegetables (mindful of potassium levels). Choose fresh meats and fish over processed varieties and store egg whites and low-phosphorus dairy alternatives.

- **Snack Selection:** Have healthy snack options readily available, like apple slices, carrot sticks, or rice cakes. Avoid high-sodium, high-potassium, or high-phosphorus snacks.

KITCHEN TOOLS FOR HEALTHY COOKING

- **Measuring Tools:** Accurate measuring cups and spoons and a kitchen scale are essential for managing portion sizes and ingredient quantities, which are crucial in a renal diet.

- **Cookware and Utensils:** Invest in quality non-stick cookware to reduce the need for cooking oils. A variety of pots and pans will facilitate cooking a range of dishes. Include tools like colanders for draining canned vegetables to remove excess sodium.

- **Blenders and Processors:** These are useful for making smoothies, soups, and purees, allowing for creative ways to include kidney-friendly ingredients in your diet.

ORGANIZING FOR CONVENIENCE AND MOTIVATION

- **Arrange for Ease of Use:** Organize your kitchen so healthy foods and tools are easily accessible. This helps in making better food choices and simplifies meal preparation.

- **Labeling for Clarity:** Consider labeling shelves or containers with notes on potassium, phosphorus, and sodium content, especially if you share your kitchen with others who might not be on a renal diet.

- **Create a Cooking-Friendly Environment:** Ensure your kitchen is pleasant and inviting. Being comfortable in your kitchen encourages cooking at home, which is often healthier than eating out.

INCORPORATING TECHNOLOGY

Apps and Resources: Use smartphone apps or online resources to track nutrition, find kidney-friendly recipes, or learn cooking techniques that suit a renal diet.

CONCLUSION

Setting up a kidney-friendly kitchen is about more than just food choices; it's about creating an environment that supports your health goals. By organizing and equipping your kitchen appropriately, you can make meal preparation more accessible, enjoyable, and aligned with your renal dietary needs.

Reading and Understanding Nutrition Labels

Correctly interpreting food labels is essential for making informed dietary choices, especially when monitoring the intake of critical nutrients such as sodium, potassium, phosphorus, and protein.

BREAKING DOWN A NUTRITION LABEL

- **Serving Size and Servings Per Container:** Consider the serving size and the number of servings per container. This information is crucial for understanding how much of each nutrient you will consume if you eat a portion of that food.
- **Calories:** While not specific to renal health, being aware of calorie intake is essential for overall health and weight management.
- **Nutrients to Limit:** Consider sodium, potassium, and phosphorus levels. These are typically listed in milligrams (mg). Choosing foods with lower nutrients is essential for a renal diet.
- **Understanding % Daily Value (%DV):** The %DV shows how much a nutrient in a serving contributes to a daily diet. A lower %DV is preferable for those on a renal diet for nutrients like sodium, potassium, and phosphorus.

IDENTIFYING HIDDEN SODIUM, POTASSIUM, AND PHOSPHORUS

- **Sodium:** Apart from the obvious sources like salt, look for terms like sodium bicarbonate (baking soda), monosodium glutamate (MSG), or any ingredient with "sodium" in its name.
- **Potassium:** Look for ingredients like potassium chloride, a common salt substitute, or any ingredient with "potassium" in its name.
- **Phosphorus:** It's often hidden in preservatives and additives. Look for ingredients with "phos" in their names.

LEARNING TO COMPARE PRODUCTS

- **Use Nutrition Labels to Compare:** When shopping, compare the nutrition labels of similar products to choose the one that best fits within your renal diet guidelines.
- **Understand Label Claims:** Be cautious of claims like "low sodium" or "reduced fat." Check the nutrition facts to see if the product fits your dietary needs.

Portion Control and its Importance

Effective management of kidney disease involves not only the careful selection
of foods but also the control of the amount of food consumed.

MEASURING PORTIONS ACCURATELY

- **Using Measuring Tools:** Utilize measuring cups, spoons, and food scales to accurately measure portions, especially for foods high in crucial nutrients like potassium and phosphorus.
- **Visual Comparisons:** Learn to estimate serving sizes using everyday visual comparisons (e.g., a portion of meat should be about the size of a deck of cards).

TIPS FOR EFFECTIVE PORTION CONTROL

- **Mindful Eating:** Pay attention to hunger and fullness cues. Eating slowly and mindfully helps you recognize when you are full.
- **Plate Method:** Use smaller plates to reduce portion sizes naturally. Fill half the plate with vegetables, a quarter with lean protein, and a quarter with grains or starches.
- **Avoid Eating from the Package:** Serve yourself a portion on a plate or bowl instead of eating directly from the package, which can lead to overeating.
- **Pre-Portion Snacks:** Divide snacks into individual portions ahead of time to avoid the temptation of overeating at once.

INCORPORATING PORTION CONTROL INTO DAILY LIFE

Making portion control a habit involves consistent practice and awareness. Use tools and techniques routinely until they become a natural part of your eating habits.

CHAPTER 4

Eating Out: Making Smart Choices

Eating out can be enjoyable and social, but it often presents obstacles for those following a specific dietary regimen. This section provides tips and strategies for making kidney-friendly choices at restaurants and other restaurants.

PREPARATION BEFORE EATING OUT

- **Research Restaurants:** Research restaurants that offer kidney-friendly menu options before dining out. Many establishments have their menus online, allowing you to plan.

- **Know the Menu:** Familiarize yourself with menu terms. Dishes labeled as creamy, breaded, or fried are typically high in sodium and phosphorus. Opt for grilled, baked, or steamed options instead.

- **Call Ahead:** Don't hesitate to call the restaurant in advance to inquire about special dietary accommodations. Many chefs are willing to modify dishes to meet your needs.

ORDERING STRATEGIES AT RESTAURANTS

- **Request Modifications:** Ask for your meal to be prepared with less salt or without added sauces, which often contain high sodium and phosphorus levels.

- **Control Portion Sizes:** Restaurant portions can be large. Consider ordering a half portion or an appetizer as your main course. Alternatively, plan to take half of your meal home for another day.

- **Choose Beverages Wisely:** Stick to water or other low-potassium drinks. Avoid or limit alcohol and high-phosphorus beverages like colas.

- **Mind Your Sides:** Choose side dishes carefully. Opt for steamed vegetables or a salad with dressing on the side instead of fries or other high-sodium options.

DEALING WITH SPECIFIC TYPES OF CUISINE

- **Fast Food:** If fast food is your only option, choose the healthiest items, such as a grilled chicken sandwich or salad. Avoid items like burgers and fries, which are typically high in sodium and unhealthy fats.

- **Ethnic Restaurants:** Each cuisine has its challenges. For instance, in Chinese restaurants, choose steamed dishes over fried ones and ask for sauce on the side. In Italian restaurants, avoid dishes with heavy cheese and cream.

SOCIALIZING AND EATING OUT

- **Communicate with Dining Companions:** Let your friends or family know your dietary needs. This can help avoid awkward situations when ordering or choosing a restaurant.

- **Focus on the Experience:** Eating out is as much about the social experience as it is about the food. Enjoy the company and the environment.

CONCLUSION

Eating out while following a renal diet requires planning and smart choices, but it doesn't have to be daunting. These strategies allow you to enjoy dining out without compromising your kidney health.

Staying Motivated and Committed

Maintaining a specialized diet over the long term can be challenging, and motivation can fluctuate. In this section, I'm eager to share strategies with you that are designed to help maintain your inspiration and commitment to your kidney health goals.

UNDERSTANDING THE IMPORTANCE OF YOUR DIET

- **Educate Yourself:** The more you understand how a renal diet supports kidney health, the more motivated you may feel. Knowledge can empower you to make informed decisions and understand the impact of your dietary choices.
- **Set Realistic Goals:** Establish achievable dietary goals. These can be as simple as reducing sodium intake in your meals or trying a new kidney-friendly recipe each week. Achieving these small goals can provide a sense of accomplishment and encourage you to continue.

FINDING SUPPORT

- **Involve Family and Friends:** Share your journey with your loved ones. Their understanding and support can make adhering to your dietary restrictions easier, especially during social events or meals.
- **Join Support Groups:** Connecting with others on a renal diet can be incredibly motivating. Support groups, whether in person or online, can provide a platform for sharing experiences, tips, and encouragement.

OVERCOMING CHALLENGES

- **Identify and Address Barriers:** Recognize what makes sticking to your diet challenging, whether it's a busy schedule, emotional eating, or lack of variety in your meals. Finding solutions to these barriers can help you stay on track.
- **Be Kind to Yourself:** Understand that setbacks happen. If you stray from your diet, acknowledge it, learn from it, and move forward without guilt.

MAINTAINING VARIETY AND ENJOYMENT IN YOUR DIET

- **Explore New Recipes:** Trying new renal-friendly recipes can keep your meals exciting and enjoyable. This cookbook and other resources can be excellent sources of inspiration.
- **Celebrate Culinary Successes:** Take pride in successful meal preparations and enjoy the process of cooking and eating healthy.

STAYING INSPIRED

- **Track Your Progress:** Keep a journal or log of your diet and how you feel. Noticing improvements in your health or well-being can be a strong motivator.
- **Reflect on the Benefits:** Regularly remind yourself of the benefits of your renal diet, not just for your kidneys but for your overall health.

CONCLUSION

Staying motivated and committed to a renal diet is a journey that involves education, support, and self-compassion. By employing these strategies, you can maintain your focus and dedication to kidney health.

CHAPTER 5

Breakfast Recipes

Kidney Care Blueberry Smoothie

Yield: 1 serving | **Prep time:** 5 minutes | **Cook time:** 0 minutes

INGREDIENTS:

- 1/2 cup fresh or frozen blueberries (low in potassium)
- 1/2 cup low-fat Greek yogurt (low in phosphorus and potassium)
- 1/4 cup water or almond milk (low in potassium)
- 1 tablespoon honey or maple syrup (optional)
- A pinch of ground cinnamon

DIRECTIONS:

1. Place the blueberries, Greek yogurt, water or almond milk, and honey or maple syrup (if using) in a blender.
2. Blend on high speed until smooth and creamy.
3. Add a pinch of ground cinnamon and blend again for a few seconds.
4. Pour the smoothie into a glass.
5. Serve immediately for the best taste and texture.

NUTRITIONAL INFORMATION:

Calories: 120 | **Protein:** 10 g | **Carbohydrates:** 18 g | **Dietary Fiber:** 2 g | **Sugars:** 15 g | **Fat:** 1 g | **Sodium:** 45 mg | **Potassium:** 150 mg | **Phosphorus:** 100 mg

Renal Diet Renal-Friendly Apple Cinnamon Oatmeal

Yield: 1 serving | **Prep time:** 5 minutes | **Cook time:** 10 minutes

INGREDIENTS:

- 1/2 cup rolled oats
- 1 cup water
- 1 small apple, peeled and diced
- 1/4 teaspoon ground cinnamon
- 1 tablespoon honey or sugar (optional)
- 1 tablespoon chopped nuts (such as walnuts or almonds, optional)

DIRECTIONS:

1. In a small saucepan, combine the rolled oats and water. Bring to a boil over medium heat.
2. Reduce the heat to low and add the diced apple and cinnamon. Stir well.
3. Simmer for about 5-7 minutes, or until the oats are soft and the mixture has thickened.
4. Remove from heat and let it cool for a few minutes.
5. If desired, sweeten with honey or sugar. Top with chopped nuts if using.
6. Serve the oatmeal warm.

NUTRITIONAL INFORMATION:

Calories: 190 | **Protein:** 5 g | **Carbohydrates:** 38 g | **Dietary Fiber:** 5 g | **Sugars:** 15 g | **Fat:** 3 g | **Sodium:** 10 mg | **Potassium:** 150 mg | **Phosphorus:** 120 mg

Rice Porridge with Apples

Yield: 1 serving | **Prep time:** 5 minutes | **Cook time:** 25 minutes

INGREDIENTS:

- 1/4 cup white rice
- 1 cup water
- 1 small apple, peeled and grated
- 1/4 teaspoon ground cinnamon
- 1 tablespoon honey or sugar (optional)
- 1 tablespoon almond slivers or chopped nuts (optional; consider renal diet restrictions)

DIRECTIONS:

1. Rinse the white rice under cold water until the water runs clear.
2. In a small saucepan, combine the rinsed rice and water. Bring to a boil over medium heat.
3. Reduce the heat to low and simmer, stirring occasionally, until the rice is soft and the mixture has thickened, about 20 minutes.
4. Add the grated apple and cinnamon to the porridge. Stir well and cook for an additional 5 minutes.
5. Remove from heat and let it cool slightly. Sweeten with honey or sugar if desired.
6. Top with almond slivers or chopped nuts if using.
7. Serve the rice porridge warm.

NUTRITIONAL INFORMATION:

Calories: 200 | **Protein:** 3 g | **Carbohydrates:** 45 g | **Dietary Fiber:** 3 g | **Sugars:** 15 g (if honey is used) | **Fat:** 1 g (3 g with nuts) | **Sodium:** 10 mg | **Potassium:** 150 mg | **Phosphorus:** 70 mg

Low-Potassium Pancakes

Yield: 1 serving | **Prep time:** 5 minutes | **Cook time:** 10 minutes

INGREDIENTS:

- 1/2 cup all-purpose flour (low in potassium)
- 1/2 teaspoon baking powder (low sodium)
- 1 tablespoon sugar
- 1/2 cup milk (use rice milk for lower potassium)
- 1 tablespoon unsalted butter, melted
- 1 egg
- A pinch of salt
- Cooking spray or a small amount of oil for the pan

DIRECTIONS:

1. Combine the flour, baking powder, sugar, and a pinch of salt in a mixing bowl.
2. In another bowl, beat the egg and mix the milk and melted butter.
3. Add the wet and dry ingredients and stir until just combined. The batter should be slightly lumpy.
4. Heat a non-stick skillet or griddle over medium heat. Lightly coat with cooking spray or oil.
5. Pour about 1/4 cup of batter onto the skillet for each pancake. Cook until bubbles form on the surface, then flip and cook the other side until golden brown, about 2 minutes per side.
6. Serve the pancakes warm.

NUTRITIONAL INFORMATION:

Calories: 450 | **Protein:** 13 g | **Carbohydrates:** 57 g | **Dietary Fiber:** 1.5 g | **Sugars:** 16 g | **Fat:** 19 g | **Sodium:** 220 mg | **Potassium:** 235 mg | **Phosphorus:** 380 mg

Egg White Omelette with Herbs

Yield: 1 serving | **Prep time:** 5 minutes | **Cook time:** 5 minutes

INGREDIENTS:

- 3 egg whites
- 1 tablespoon water
- 1/4 teaspoon black pepper
- 1/4 cup mixed fresh herbs (such as parsley, chives, and thyme), chopped
- 1 teaspoon olive oil
- 2 tablespoons diced bell pepper (optional)
- 2 tablespoons diced onion (optional)

DIRECTIONS:

1. In a bowl, whisk together the egg whites, water, and black pepper until frothy.
2. Heat the olive oil in a non-stick skillet over medium heat.
3. If using, add the diced bell pepper and onion to the skillet, and sauté for 1-2 minutes until they soften.
4. Pour the egg white mixture into the skillet, ensuring it spreads evenly.
5. Sprinkle the chopped herbs over the top of the egg whites.
6. Cook for 2-3 minutes until the bottom sets. Carefully fold the omelet in half, then cook for another 1-2 minutes until fully set.
7. Gently slide the omelet onto a plate and serve immediately.

NUTRITIONAL INFORMATION:

Calories: 120 | **Protein:** 15 g | **Carbohydrates:** 4 g | **Dietary Fiber:** 1 g | **Sugars:** 2 g | **Fat:** 5 g | **Sodium:** 170 mg | **Potassium:** 220 mg | **Phosphorus:** 45 mg

Renal Diet Low-Sodium Scrambled Eggs

Yield: 1 serving | **Prep time:** 3 minutes | **Cook time:** 5 minutes

INGREDIENTS:

- 2 large egg whites
- 1 tablespoon milk (preferably low-fat or almond milk)
- A pinch of black pepper
- 1/2 teaspoon olive oil
- 1 tablespoon chopped fresh herbs (such as parsley or chives, optional)
- 1 tablespoon diced tomatoes (optional)

DIRECTIONS:

1. In a small bowl, whisk together egg whites, milk, and black pepper until well combined.
2. Heat olive oil in a non-stick skillet over medium heat.
3. Pour the egg mixture into the skillet. Let it sit without stirring for about 1 minute until it begins to set on the bottom.
4. Gently stir the eggs, folding them from the edge to the center. Cook for 2-3 more minutes or until fully cooked but moist.
5. If using, sprinkle with chopped herbs and diced tomatoes before serving.
6. Serve the scrambled eggs hot.

NUTRITIONAL INFORMATION:

Calories: 100 | **Protein:** 11 g | **Carbohydrates:** 2 g | **Dietary Fiber:** 0.5 g | **Sugars:** 1.5 g | **Fat:** 5 g | **Sodium:** 110 mg | **Potassium:** 200 mg | **Phosphorus:** 70 mg

Low-Sodium French Toast

Yield: 1 serving | **Prep time:** 5 minutes | **Cook time:** 10 minutes

INGREDIENTS:

- 2 slices low-sodium bread
- 1 egg
- 1/4 cup milk (preferably low-fat or almond milk)
- 1/4 teaspoon vanilla extract
- 1/4 teaspoon ground cinnamon
- 1 teaspoon unsalted butter or cooking spray
- 1 tablespoon maple syrup or honey (optional)
- Fresh berries or sliced fruit for topping (optional)

DIRECTIONS:

1. Whisk the egg, milk, vanilla extract, and cinnamon in a shallow bowl.
2. Dip each slice of bread into the egg mixture, ensuring both sides are well coated.
3. Heat a non-stick skillet over medium heat. Add the unsalted butter or coat with cooking spray.
4. Place the soaked bread slices in the skillet. Cook for 4-5 minutes on each side until golden brown is cooked.
5. Transfer the French toast to a plate.
6. Top with maple syrup or honey and fresh berries or sliced fruit, if desired.
7. Serve warm.

NUTRITIONAL INFORMATION:

Calories: 250 | **Protein:** 12 g | **Carbohydrates:** 35 g | **Dietary Fiber:** 2 g | **Sugars:** 12 g (if using maple syrup) | **Fat:** 8 g | **Sodium:** 200 mg | **Potassium:** 200 mg | **Phosphorus:** 180 mg

Berry and Almond Yogurt Parfait

Yield: 1 serving | **Prep time:** 5 minutes | **Cook time:** 0 minutes

INGREDIENTS:

- 1/2 cup low-fat Greek yogurt (low in phosphorus)
- 1/4 cup fresh blueberries
- 1/4 cup fresh strawberries, sliced
- 1 tablespoon almond slivers (optional; consider renal diet restrictions)
- 1 teaspoon honey or maple syrup (optional)

DIRECTIONS:

1. Layer half of the Greek yogurt at the bottom in a serving glass or bowl.
2. Add a layer of half of the blueberries and strawberries.
3. Repeat the layers with the remaining yogurt and berries.
4. If using, sprinkle almond slivers on top for added crunch.
5. Drizzle with honey or maple syrup, if desired.
6. Serve immediately to enjoy the freshness of the berries and the creaminess of the yogurt.

NUTRITIONAL INFORMATION:

Calories: 150 | **Protein:** 12 g | **Carbohydrates:** 18 g | **Dietary Fiber:** 2 g | **Sugars:** 15 g | **Fat:** 4 g (6 g with almonds) | **Sodium:** 45 mg | **Potassium:** 250 mg | **Phosphorus:** 150 mg

Kidney-Friendly Banana Bread

Yield: 1 serving | **Prep time:** 15 minutes | **Cook time:** 30 minutes

INGREDIENTS:

- 1/2 ripe banana, mashed
- 1 tablespoon unsalted butter, softened
- 2 tablespoons sugar
- 1 egg
- 1/4 cup all-purpose flour
- 1/8 teaspoon baking powder (low sodium)
- 1/8 teaspoon baking soda
- A pinch of salt
- 1/8 teaspoon vanilla extract
- 1 tablespoon chopped walnuts or pecans (optional; consider renal diet restrictions)

DIRECTIONS:

1. Preheat your oven to 350°F (175°C). Grease a small loaf pan.
2. Combine the mashed banana with the softened butter and sugar in a mixing bowl. Beat until well mixed.
3. Add the egg and vanilla extract to the banana mixture and beat until smooth.
4. Sift the flour, baking powder, baking soda, and a pinch of salt in a separate bowl.
5. Gradually add the dry ingredients to the banana mixture, stirring until incorporated.
6. If using, fold in the chopped nuts.
7. Pour the batter into the prepared loaf pan. Smooth the top with a spatula.
8. Bake in the oven for about 30 minutes or until a toothpick inserted into the center comes clean.
9. Remove it from the oven and let it cool in the pan for 10 minutes, then transfer it to a wire rack to cool completely.
10. Slice and serve the banana bread.

NUTRITIONAL INFORMATION:

Calories: 400 | **Protein:** 7 g | **Carbohydrates:** 58 g | **Dietary Fiber:** 2 g | **Sugars:** 30 g | **Fat:** 16 g (18 g with nuts) | **Sodium:** 150 mg | **Potassium:** 250 mg | **Phosphorus:** 100 mg

Kidney Care Fruit Salad

Yield: 1 serving | **Prep time:** 10 minutes | **Cook time:** 0 minutes

INGREDIENTS:

- 1/4 cup sliced strawberries
- 1/4 cup blueberries
- 1/4 cup diced pineapple (canned in juice, not syrup, and drained)
- 1/4 apple, cored and chopped
- A squeeze of fresh lemon juice
- 1 teaspoon honey (optional)

DIRECTIONS:

1. Combine the sliced strawberries, blueberries, diced pineapple, and chopped apple in a medium-sized bowl.
2. Squeeze fresh lemon juice over the fruit mixture. This adds flavor and helps keep the fruits, especially the apple, from browning.
3. Drizzle honey over the fruit for added sweetness, if desired.
4. Gently toss all the ingredients together until well-mixed.
5. Serve immediately, or refrigerate for up to an hour before serving to allow the flavors to meld together.

NUTRITIONAL INFORMATION:

Calories: 100 | **Protein:** 1 g | **Carbohydrates:** 25 g | **Dietary Fiber:** 3 g | **Sugars:** 20 g | **Fat:** 0 g | **Sodium:** 5 mg | **Potassium:** 150 mg | **Phosphorus:** 20 mg

Carrot and Zucchini Muffins
(Low-Potassium)

Yield: 1 serving | **Prep time:** 15 minutes | **Cook time:** 20 minutes

INGREDIENTS:

- 1/4 cup grated carrot
- 1/4 cup grated zucchini, excess moisture squeezed out
- 1/2 cup all-purpose flour
- 1/4 teaspoon baking powder (low sodium)
- 1/4 teaspoon baking soda
- A pinch of salt
- 1/4 teaspoon cinnamon
- 1 tablespoon unsalted butter, melted
- 2 tablespoons sugar
- 1/4 egg, beaten (about one tablespoon of beaten egg)
- 1 tablespoon low-fat milk
- 1/4 teaspoon vanilla extract

DIRECTIONS:

1. Preheat your oven to 350°F (175°C). Grease a muffin cup in a muffin tin.
2. In a small bowl, combine the grated carrot and zucchini.
3. Mix the flour, baking powder, baking soda, salt, and cinnamon in another bowl.
4. Whisk the melted butter, sugar, beaten egg, milk, and vanilla extract in a separate bowl.
5. Add the wet ingredients to the dry ingredients, stirring until combined.
6. Fold in the grated carrot and zucchini.
7. Spoon the batter into the prepared muffin cup.
8. Bake in the preheated oven for 20 minutes or until a toothpick inserted into the center of the muffin comes out clean.
9. Allow the muffin to cool in the pan for a few minutes, then transfer to a wire rack to cool completely.

NUTRITIONAL INFORMATION:

Calories: 320 | **Protein:** 5 g | **Carbohydrates:** 50 g | **Dietary Fiber:** 2 g | **Sugars:** 20 g | **Fat:** 11 g | **Sodium:** 150 mg | **Potassium:** 150 mg | **Phosphorus:** 100 mg

Baked Apples with Cinnamon

Yield: 1 serving | **Prep time:** 5 minutes | **Cook time:** 30 minutes

INGREDIENTS:

- 1 medium apple, cored and sliced
- 1/4 teaspoon ground cinnamon
- 1 teaspoon honey or brown sugar (optional)
- A splash of water

DIRECTIONS:

1. Preheat your oven to 350°F (175°C).
2. Place the sliced apple in a small baking dish.
3. Sprinkle the apple slices evenly with ground cinnamon. Drizzle with honey or sprinkle with brown sugar, if desired.
4. Add a splash of water to the bottom of the dish (just enough to cover the base).
5. Cover the dish with aluminum foil and bake in the oven for 25-30 minutes or until the apples are soft and tender.
6. Carefully remove from the oven, uncover, and allow to cool slightly.
7. If desired, Serve the baked apples warm, perhaps with a dollop of low-phosphorus whipped cream or yogurt.

NUTRITIONAL INFORMATION:

Calories: 80 (95 with honey) | **Protein:** 0.5 g | **Carbohydrates:** 22 g (25 g with honey) | **Dietary Fiber:** 4 g | **Sugars:** 16 g (19 g with honey) | **Fat:** 0 g | **Sodium:** 2 mg | **Potassium:** 150 mg | **Phosphorus:** 10 mg

Low-Phosphorus Muesli

Yield: 1 serving | **Prep time:** 5 minutes | **Cook time:** 0 minutes

INGREDIENTS:

- 1/3 cup rolled oats
- 1/4 cup rice milk or almond milk
- 1 tablespoon honey or maple syrup
- 1/4 apple, cored and grated
- 1 tablespoon raisins
- A pinch of cinnamon

DIRECTIONS:

1. Combine the rolled oats, rice, or almond milk in a bowl. Stir well.
2. Add the grated apple and raisins to the oat mixture.
3. Drizzle with honey or maple syrup.
4. Sprinkle a pinch of cinnamon over the top for flavor.
5. Stir all the ingredients together until well combined.
6. Cover the bowl and refrigerate overnight, or for at least 1 hour, to allow the oats to soften and flavors to meld.
7. Serve chilled. You can add a splash of milk if the muesli is too thick.

NUTRITIONAL INFORMATION:

Calories: 240 | **Protein:** 5 g | **Carbohydrates:** 50 g | **Dietary Fiber:** 4 g | **Sugars:** 22 g | **Fat:** 3 g | **Sodium:** 30 mg | **Potassium:** 200 mg | **Phosphorus:** 90 mg

Egg Whites and Spinach Wrap

Yield: 1 serving | **Prep time:** 5 minutes | **Cook time:** 10 minutes

INGREDIENTS:

- 3 egg whites
- 1/2 cup fresh spinach, chopped
- 1 low-sodium whole wheat tortilla
- 1 tablespoon shredded low-sodium cheese (optional)
- 1 teaspoon olive oil
- A pinch of black pepper
- A pinch of garlic powder

DIRECTIONS:

1. Heat olive oil in a non-stick skillet over medium heat.
2. Whisk the egg whites, black pepper, and garlic powder in a bowl.
3. Pour the egg whites into the skillet and cook for about 2 minutes until they begin to set.
4. Add the chopped spinach to the egg whites and continue to cook until the spinach wilts and the egg whites are fully cooked, about 2-3 more minutes.
5. Warm the tortilla in a separate pan or the microwave for a few seconds.
6. Place the cooked egg whites and spinach in the center of the tortilla. Sprinkle with shredded cheese if using.
7. Fold the tortilla to wrap the egg whites and spinach.
8. Serve the wrap warm.

NUTRITIONAL INFORMATION:

Calories: 180 | **Protein:** 18 g | **Carbohydrates:** 15 g | **Dietary Fiber:** 2 g | **Sugars:** 1 g | **Fat:** 6 g | **Sodium:** 200 mg | **Potassium:** 220 mg | **Phosphorus:** 100 mg

Low-Potassium Bagel with Cream Cheese

Yield: 1 serving | **Prep time:** 2 minutes | **Cook time:** 0 minutes

INGREDIENTS:

- 1 low-potassium bagel (such as white or sourdough)
- 2 tablespoons low-fat cream cheese

DIRECTIONS:

1. Slice the bagel in half horizontally.
2. Toast the bagel halves to your desired level of crispiness.
3. Spread one tablespoon of low-fat cream cheese evenly on each half of the bagel.
4. If desired, add a sprinkle of herbs like dill or chives for extra flavor.
5. Serve the bagel halves open-faced or sandwich them together.
6. Enjoy your renal diet-friendly bagel as a quick breakfast or snack.

NUTRITIONAL INFORMATION:

Calories: 260 | **Protein:** 11 g | **Carbohydrates:** 48 g | **Dietary Fiber:** 2 g | **Sugars:** 6 g | **Fat:** 4 g | **Sodium:** 360 mg | **Potassium:** 90 mg | **Phosphorus:** 100 mg

Pineapple Rice Pudding

(with low-potassium pineapples)

Yield: 1 serving | **Prep time:** 5 minutes | **Cook time:** 25 minutes

INGREDIENTS:

- 1/4 cup uncooked white rice
- 1 cup water
- 1/2 cup low-fat milk
- 1/4 cup canned low-potassium pineapple chunks, drained
- 1 tablespoon sugar
- 1/4 teaspoon vanilla extract
- A pinch of cinnamon (optional)

DIRECTIONS:

1. In a small saucepan, bring water to a boil. Add rice and reduce heat to a simmer. Cover and cook until rice is tender, about 20 minutes.
2. Stir in milk, pineapple chunks, and sugar. Cook on low heat for another 5 minutes, stirring occasionally.
3. Remove from heat and stir in vanilla extract. Add a pinch of cinnamon if desired.
4. Let the rice pudding cool for a few minutes. It will thicken as it cools.
5. Serve warm or chill in the refrigerator if you prefer it cold.
6. Garnish with a sprinkle of cinnamon before serving, if desired.

NUTRITIONAL INFORMATION:

Calories: 220 | **Protein:** 5 g | **Carbohydrates:** 45 g | **Dietary Fiber:** 1 g | **Sugars:** 20 g | **Fat:** 2 g | **Sodium:** 50 mg | **Potassium:** 120 mg | **Phosphorus:** 100 mg

Renal-Friendly Cranberry Muffins

Yield: 1 serving | **Prep time:** 10 minutes | **Cook time:** 20 minutes

INGREDIENTS:

- 1/4 cup all-purpose flour
- 1 tablespoon sugar
- 1/4 teaspoon baking powder (low sodium)
- 1/8 teaspoon baking soda
- A pinch of salt
- 1 tablespoon unsalted butter, melted
- 2 tablespoons low-fat milk
- 1/4 egg, beaten (about one tablespoon of beaten egg)
- 1/4 teaspoon vanilla extract
- 2 tablespoons dried cranberries (lower in potassium than fresh)

DIRECTIONS:

1. Preheat your oven to 375°F (190°C). Grease a muffin cup in a muffin tin.
2. Mix the flour, sugar, baking powder, baking soda, and salt in a small bowl.
3. Combine the melted butter, milk, beaten egg, and vanilla extract in another bowl.
4. Add the wet and dry ingredients and stir until just combined.
5. Gently fold in the dried cranberries.
6. Spoon the batter into the greased muffin cup.
7. Bake in the preheated oven for 20 minutes or until a toothpick inserted into the center of the muffin comes out clean.
8. Allow the muffin to cool in the pan for a few minutes, then transfer to a wire rack to cool completely.

NUTRITIONAL INFORMATION:

Calories: 230 | **Protein:** 3 g | **Carbohydrates:** 35 g | **Dietary Fiber:** 1 g | **Sugars:** 15 g | **Fat:** 9 g | **Sodium:** 75 mg | **Potassium:** 60 mg | **Phosphorus:** 90 mg

Savory Oatmeal with Egg Whites

Yield: 1 serving | **Prep time:** 5 minutes | **Cook time:** 10 minutes

INGREDIENTS:

- 1/2 cup rolled oats
- 1 cup water
- 2 egg whites
- A pinch of black pepper
- 1 tablespoon chopped green onions
- 1 teaspoon olive oil
- 1 tablespoon grated low-sodium cheese (optional)
- A pinch of garlic powder (optional)

DIRECTIONS:

1. In a small saucepan, bring water to a boil. Add the oats and cook over medium heat for about 5 minutes, until the oats are soft and the water is absorbed.
2. While cooking oats, whisk the egg whites with black pepper and garlic powder (if using) in a bowl.
3. Heat olive oil in a non-stick skillet over medium heat. Add the egg whites and scramble until fully cooked, about 3 minutes.
4. Stir the scrambled egg whites and chopped green onions into the cooked oatmeal.
5. Top with grated low-sodium cheese, if desired.
6. Serve the savory oatmeal hot, seasoned with additional black pepper to taste.

NUTRITIONAL INFORMATION:

Calories: 220 | **Protein:** 13 g | **Carbohydrates:** 27 g | **Dietary Fiber:** 4 g | **Sugars:** 1 g | **Fat:** 7 g (8 g with cheese) | **Sodium:** 100 mg | **Potassium:** 150 mg | **Phosphorus:** 150 mg

Kidney Diet-Friendly Pancakes with Apple Sauce

Yield: 1 serving | **Prep time:** 10 minutes | **Cook time:** 10 minutes

INGREDIENTS:

- 1/2 cup all-purpose flour
- 1/2 teaspoon baking powder (low sodium)
- 1 tablespoon sugar
- 1/2 cup low-fat milk
- 1 egg
- 1 tablespoon unsalted butter, melted
- Cooking spray or a small amount of oil for the pan
- 1/4 cup low-potassium apple sauce (homemade or store-bought)

DIRECTIONS:

1. Mix the flour, baking powder, and sugar in a medium bowl.
2. In a separate bowl, beat the egg and mix the milk and melted butter.
3. Gradually add the wet and dry ingredients, stirring until combined. Avoid over-mixing to keep the pancakes light and fluffy.
4. Heat a non-stick skillet over medium heat. Lightly coat with cooking spray or oil.
5. Pour about 1/4 cup of batter per pancake onto the skillet. Cook until bubbles form on the surface, then flip and cook the other side until golden brown, about 2 minutes per side.
6. Serve the pancakes warm, topped with the apple sauce.

NUTRITIONAL INFORMATION:

Calories: 420 | **Protein:** 11 g | **Carbohydrates:** 60 g | **Dietary Fiber:** 2 g | **Sugars:** 20 g | **Fat:** 16 g | **Sodium:** 200 mg | **Potassium:** 250 mg | **Phosphorus:** 290 mg

Renal Diet Veggie Frittata

Yield: 1 serving | **Prep time:** 10 minutes | **Cook time:** 15 minutes

INGREDIENTS:

- 3 egg whites
- 1/4 cup diced bell pepper (red or green)
- 1/4 cup diced onion
- 1/4 cup chopped fresh spinach
- 1/2 teaspoon olive oil
- A pinch of black pepper
- A pinch of garlic powder
- 1 tablespoon shredded low-sodium cheese (optional)

DIRECTIONS:

1. Preheat the oven to 375°F (190°C).

2. Heat olive oil in an oven-safe non-stick skillet over medium heat. Add diced bell pepper, onion, and sauté for 2-3 minutes until softened.

3. Stir in the chopped spinach and cook for an additional minute.

4. Whisk the egg whites, black pepper, and garlic powder in a bowl.

5. Pour the egg mixture into the skillet over the vegetables. Cook without stirring for about 2 minutes until the edges start to set.

6. Sprinkle with shredded cheese if using. Then, transfer the skillet to the preheated oven.

7. Bake 10-12 minutes until the frittata is set and lightly golden on top.

8. Remove from the oven, let it cool slightly, then slide it onto a plate and serve.

NUTRITIONAL INFORMATION:

Calories: 120 | **Protein:** 14 g | **Carbohydrates:** 6 g | **Dietary Fiber:** 1 g | **Sugars:** 3 g | **Fat:** 5 g (6 g with cheese) | **Sodium:** 150 mg | **Potassium:** 220 mg | **Phosphorus:** 90 mg

Kidney-Friendly Smoothie Bowl

Yield: 1 serving | **Prep time:** 5 minutes | **Cook time:** 0 minutes

INGREDIENTS:

- 1/2 cup fresh or frozen blueberries (low in potassium)
- 1/2 banana, sliced
- 1/2 cup rice milk or almond milk
- 1/4 cup low-fat Greek yogurt (low in phosphorus)
- 1 tablespoon honey or maple syrup
- 1 tablespoon ground flaxseed (optional)

DIRECTIONS:

1. Combine the blueberries, banana, rice milk, almond milk, and Greek yogurt in a blender.

2. Blend until smooth and creamy. Add more milk to reach your desired consistency if the mixture is too thick.

3. Pour the smoothie into a bowl.

4. Drizzle with honey or maple syrup.

5. Sprinkle ground flaxseed on top for added fiber if using.

6. Serve immediately and enjoy your nutrient-packed, kidney-friendly smoothie bowl.

NUTRITIONAL INFORMATION:

Calories: 240 | **Protein:** 10 g | **Carbohydrates:** 45 g | **Dietary Fiber:** 4 g | **Sugars:** 30 g | **Fat:** 3 g | **Sodium:** 50 mg | **Potassium:** 300 mg | **Phosphorus:** 100 mg

Creamy Polenta with Fresh Berries

Yield: 1 serving | **Prep time:** 5 minutes | **Cook time:** 20 minutes

INGREDIENTS:

- 1/4 cup polenta (cornmeal)
- 1 cup water
- A pinch of salt
- 1/4 cup low-fat milk or almond milk
- 1/2 tablespoon unsalted butter or margarine
- 1/2 cup mixed fresh berries (such as blueberries, raspberries, and strawberries)
- 1 teaspoon honey or sugar (optional)

DIRECTIONS:

1. In a small saucepan, bring water to a boil. Gradually add the polenta and salt, stirring constantly.
2. Reduce the heat to low and continue to cook, stirring frequently, until the polenta thickens and becomes creamy, about 15-20 minutes.
3. Remove from heat and stir in the milk, butter, or margarine until well combined and smooth.
4. Transfer the polenta to a serving bowl.
5. Top with fresh berries and drizzle with honey or sugar, if desired.
6. Serve warm, enjoying the contrast of the creamy polenta with the fresh, juicy berries.

NUTRITIONAL INFORMATION:

Calories: 210 | **Protein:** 5 g | **Carbohydrates:** 37 g | **Dietary Fiber:** 3 g | **Sugars:** 8 g (9 g if honey is used) | **Fat:** 5 g | **Sodium:** 65 mg | **Potassium:** 150 mg | **Phosphorus:** 100 mg

Pearled Barley with Cinnamon and Nutmeg

Yield: 1 serving | **Prep time:** 5 minutes | **Cook time:** 25 minutes

INGREDIENTS:

- 1/4 cup pearled barley
- 1 cup water
- A pinch of cinnamon
- A pinch of nutmeg
- 1 teaspoon honey or sugar (optional)

DIRECTIONS:

1. Rinse the pearled barley under cold water until the water runs clear.
2. In a small saucepan, combine the rinsed barley and water. Bring to a boil.
3. Reduce heat to low, cover, and simmer for about 25 minutes until the barley is tender and most water is absorbed.
4. Remove from heat and let it stand covered for 5 minutes.
5. Fluff the barley with a fork and stir in a pinch of cinnamon and nutmeg.
6. Sweeten with honey or sugar if desired.
7. Serve warm as a side dish or a healthy snack.

NUTRITIONAL INFORMATION:

Calories: 160 | **Protein:** 3 g | **Carbohydrates:** 35 g | **Dietary Fiber:** 6 g | **Sugars:** 5 g (if honey is used) | **Fat:** 1 g | **Sodium:** 5 mg | **Potassium:** 85 mg | **Phosphorus:** 60 mg

Egg Salad on Toast
(using low-sodium bread)

Yield: 1 serving | **Prep time:** 5 minutes | **Cook time:** 10 minutes

---

INGREDIENTS:

- 2 eggs
- 1 tablespoon low-fat mayonnaise
- A pinch of black pepper
- A pinch of paprika (optional)
- 1 slice of low-sodium bread
- A few lettuce leaves (optional)

DIRECTIONS:

1. Place the eggs in a saucepan and cover with cold water. Bring to a boil, then reduce heat and simmer for 10 minutes.
2. Remove eggs from heat, cool them under cold running water, and peel them.
3. In a bowl, chop the hard-boiled eggs and mix with low-fat mayonnaise, black pepper, and paprika (if using).
4. Toast the slice of low-sodium bread to your desired crispiness.
5. Spread the egg salad evenly on top of the toasted bread.
6. Add a few lettuce leaves to the egg salad if desired.
7. Serve immediately.

NUTRITIONAL INFORMATION:

Calories: 280 | **Protein:** 14 g | **Carbohydrates:** 20 g | **Dietary Fiber:** 2 g | **Sugars:** 3 g | **Fat:** 15 g | **Sodium:** 200 mg | **Potassium:** 180 mg | **Phosphorus:** 220 mg

Baked Peach Oatmeal

Yield: 1 serving | **Prep time:** 5 minutes | **Cook time:** 20 minutes

---

INGREDIENTS:

- 1/2 cup rolled oats
- 3/4 cup water or almond milk
- 1 small peach, sliced
- 1 tablespoon honey or maple syrup
- 1/4 teaspoon cinnamon
- A pinch of nutmeg
- 1 tablespoon chopped almonds (optional)

DIRECTIONS:

1. Preheat your oven to 375°F (190°C).
2. Combine the rolled oats and water or almond milk in a small baking dish.
3. Arrange the peach slices on top of the oats.
4. Drizzle the honey or maple syrup over the peaches and oats.
5. Sprinkle with cinnamon and nutmeg.
6. Bake in the oven for 20 minutes or until the oats are cooked and the peaches are tender.
7. If desired, sprinkle chopped almonds on top after baking.
8. Serve warm.

NUTRITIONAL INFORMATION:

Calories: 250 | **Protein:** 6 g | **Carbohydrates:** 45 g | **Dietary Fiber:** 5 g | **Sugars:** 20 g | **Fat:** 5 g (7 g with almonds) | **Sodium:** 30 mg | **Potassium:** 250 mg | **Phosphorus:** 120 mg

Grilled Bell Peppers and Egg Whites

Yield: 1 serving | **Prep time:** 5 minutes | **Cook time:** 10 minutes

INGREDIENTS:

- 1/2 bell pepper, sliced (red or green for lower potassium)
- 3 egg whites
- 1 teaspoon olive oil
- A pinch of black pepper
- A pinch of garlic powder

DIRECTIONS:

1. Heat olive oil in a grill pan or skillet over medium heat.
2. Add the sliced bell peppers to the pan and grill them on each side for 3-4 minutes until they are slightly charred and tender.
3. Whisk together the egg whites with black pepper and garlic powder in a bowl.
4. In another non-stick skillet, pour the egg whites and cook over medium heat for about 2 minutes until the bottom sets.
5. Carefully fold the omelet in half and cook for another 2 minutes until fully set.
6. Serve the grilled bell peppers alongside or on the egg whites omelet.

NUTRITIONAL INFORMATION:

Calories: 130 | **Protein:** 14 g | **Carbohydrates:** 5 g | **Dietary Fiber:** 1 g | **Sugars:** 3 g | **Fat:** 5 g | **Sodium:** 150 mg | **Potassium:** 200 mg | **Phosphorus:** 45 mg

Low-Phosphorus Cheese Omelette

Yield: 1 serving | **Prep time:** 5 minutes | **Cook time:** 5 minutes

INGREDIENTS:

- 2 large eggs
- 2 tablespoons water
- A pinch of black pepper
- 1 teaspoon unsalted butter or olive oil
- 1/4 cup shredded low-phosphorus cheese (like Swiss or mozzarella)
- 1 tablespoon chopped chives or green onions (optional)

DIRECTIONS:

1. Whisk the eggs, water, and black pepper in a bowl until well combined.
2. Heat the butter or olive oil in a non-stick skillet over medium heat.
3. Pour the egg mixture into the skillet. Let it cook without stirring for about 1 minute until the bottom starts to set.
4. Sprinkle the shredded cheese and chopped chives or green onions over the egg.
5. Gently fold one side of the omelet over the cheese. Cook for another 2-3 minutes or until the cheese melts and the egg is cooked to your liking.
6. Carefully slide the omelet onto a plate and serve immediately.

NUTRITIONAL INFORMATION:

Calories: 250 | **Protein:** 18 g | **Carbohydrates:** 2 g | **Dietary Fiber:** 0 g | **Sugars:** 1 g | **Fat:** 18 g | **Sodium:** 220 mg | **Potassium:** 200 mg | **Phosphorus:** 150 mg

Banana and Blueberry Pancakes

Yield: 1 serving | **Prep time:** 10 minutes | **Cook time:** 10 minutes

INGREDIENTS:

- 1/2 ripe banana, mashed
- 1/4 cup all-purpose flour
- 1/2 teaspoon baking powder (low sodium)
- 1/4 cup low-fat milk
- 1 egg
- 1/4 cup fresh or frozen blueberries
- 1 teaspoon unsalted butter or cooking spray
- 1 tablespoon honey or maple syrup (optional)

DIRECTIONS:

1. Combine the mashed banana with the egg and milk in a mixing bowl. Stir until well mixed.

2. In a separate bowl, mix the flour and baking powder.

3. Gradually add the dry ingredients to the banana mixture, stirring until combined. Avoid over-mixing to keep the pancakes light.

4. Gently fold the blueberries into the batter.

5. Heat a non-stick skillet over medium heat and coat with unsalted butter or cooking spray.

6. Pour about 1/4 cup of batter per pancake onto the skillet. Cook until bubbles form on the surface, then flip and cook the other side until golden brown, about 2 minutes per side.

7. Serve the pancakes warm, drizzled with honey or maple syrup if desired.

NUTRITIONAL INFORMATION:

Calories: 320 | **Protein:** 10 g | **Carbohydrates:** 55 g | **Dietary Fiber:** 3 g | **Sugars:** 25 g | **Fat:** 8 g | **Sodium:** 200 mg | **Potassium:** 300 mg | **Phosphorus:** 150 mg

Chia Seed Pudding with Berries

Yield: 1 serving | **Prep time:** 5 minutes | **Cook time:** 0 minutes
(requires refrigeration for at least 2 hours or overnight)

INGREDIENTS:

- 2 tablespoons chia seeds
- 1/2 cup almond milk (or another low-potassium milk alternative)
- 1/2 teaspoon vanilla extract
- 1 teaspoon honey or maple syrup (optional)
- 1/4 cup fresh berries (such as blueberries or strawberries)

DIRECTIONS:

1. Combine the chia seeds and almond milk in a small bowl or jar. Stir well.

2. Add the vanilla extract and honey or maple syrup, if using, and mix thoroughly.

3. Cover the bowl or jar and refrigerate for at least 2 hours or overnight until the chia seeds have absorbed the liquid and the mixture has a pudding-like consistency.

4. Once set, remove it from the refrigerator and give it a good stir.

5. Top the chia pudding with fresh berries before serving.

6. Enjoy a healthy and kidney-friendly breakfast or snack.

NUTRITIONAL INFORMATION:

Calories: 180 | **Protein:** 5 g | **Carbohydrates:** 24 g | **Dietary Fiber:** 10 g | **Sugars:** 8 g | **Fat:** 8 g | **Sodium:** 50 mg | **Potassium:** 150 mg | **Phosphorus:** 200 mg

Low-Sodium Veggie Breakfast Hash

Yield: 1 serving | **Prep time:** 10 minutes | **Cook time:** 15 minutes

INGREDIENTS:

- 1/2 cup diced potatoes
- 1/4 cup diced bell peppers (red or green)
- 1/4 cup diced onion
- 1/4 cup chopped fresh spinach
- 1 tablespoon olive oil
- A pinch of black pepper
- A pinch of garlic powder
- 1 egg (optional)

DIRECTIONS:

1. Heat the olive oil in a non-stick skillet over medium heat.
2. Add the diced potatoes to the skillet and cook for about 5 minutes or until they soften.
3. Add the diced bell peppers and onion to the skillet with the potatoes. Continue cooking for another 5 minutes, stirring occasionally, until the vegetables are tender and slightly browned.
4. Stir in the chopped spinach, black pepper, and garlic powder. Cook for an additional 2 minutes.
5. If desired, create a small well in the center of the hash and crack an egg into it. Cover the skillet and cook until the egg white is set but the yolk is still runny after about 4 minutes.
6. Serve the veggie hash hot, with the egg on top if you included it.

NUTRITIONAL INFORMATION:

Calories: 250 (300 with egg) | **Protein:** 4 g (9 g with egg) | **Carbohydrates:** 23 g | **Dietary Fiber:** 3 g | **Sugars:** 4 g | **Fat:** 16 g (20 g with egg) | **Sodium:** 50 mg | **Potassium:** 450 mg | **Phosphorus:** 100 mg (170 mg with egg)

Apple and Walnut Salad

Yield: 1 serving | **Prep time:** 10 minutes | **Cook time:** 0 minutes

INGREDIENTS:

- 1 small apple, cored and chopped
- 1 tablespoon chopped walnuts (consider renal diet restrictions)
- 1 cup mixed salad greens
- 1 tablespoon low-fat feta cheese, crumbled
- 1 teaspoon olive oil
- 1 teaspoon balsamic vinegar
- A pinch of black pepper

DIRECTIONS:

1. Combine the chopped apple, salad greens, and chopped walnuts in a salad bowl.
2. Sprinkle the crumbled feta cheese over the salad.
3. Whisk the olive oil and balsamic vinegar in a small bowl. Drizzle this dressing over the salad.
4. Toss the salad gently to coat everything evenly with the dressing.
5. Season with a pinch of black pepper to taste.
6. Serve the salad immediately, fresh and crisp.

NUTRITIONAL INFORMATION:

Calories: 200 | **Protein:** 4 g | **Carbohydrates:** 20 g | **Dietary Fiber:** 3 g | **Sugars:** 12 g | **Fat:** 12 g | **Sodium:** 150 mg | **Potassium:** 200 mg | **Phosphorus:** 70 mg

Tofu Scramble with Vegetables

Yield: 1 serving | **Prep time:** 10 minutes | **Cook time:** 10 minutes

INGREDIENTS:

- 1/2 block (about 7 oz) firm tofu, drained and crumbled
- 1/4 cup diced bell peppers (red or green)
- 1/4 cup diced onion
- 1/4 cup chopped fresh spinach
- 1 teaspoon olive oil
- 1/4 teaspoon turmeric (for color)
- A pinch of black pepper
- A pinch of garlic powder
- 1 tablespoon nutritional yeast (optional for a cheesy flavor)

DIRECTIONS:

1. Heat olive oil in a non-stick skillet over medium heat.
2. Add diced bell peppers and onions to the skillet and sauté for 3-4 minutes until they soften.
3. Crumble the tofu into the skillet. Add turmeric, black pepper, and garlic powder. Stir well to combine and cook for about 5 minutes, until the tofu is heated and slightly browned.
4. Stir in the chopped spinach and cook for another minute until it wilts.
5. If using, sprinkle nutritional yeast over the scramble and mix well.
6. Serve the tofu scramble hot.

NUTRITIONAL INFORMATION:

Calories: 200 | **Protein:** 18 g | **Carbohydrates:** 10 g | **Dietary Fiber:** 3 g | **Sugars:** 3 g | **Fat:** 10 g | **Sodium:** 60 mg | **Potassium:** 300 mg | **Phosphorus:** 200 mg

Low-Potassium Potato Pancakes

Yield: 1 serving | **Prep time:** 10 minutes | **Cook time:** 15 minutes

INGREDIENTS:

- 1 small potato, peeled and grated
- 1 tablespoon onion, finely chopped
- 1 egg white
- 1 tablespoon all-purpose flour
- A pinch of black pepper
- 1 teaspoon olive oil

DIRECTIONS:

1. After grating the potato, place it in a clean cloth and squeeze out as much liquid as possible. This step is essential to ensure crispy pancakes.
2. Mix the grated potato, chopped onion, egg white, flour, and black pepper until well combined.
3. Heat the olive oil in a non-stick skillet over medium heat.
4. Scoop the potato mixture into the skillet, forming small pancakes. Flatten them slightly with a spatula.
5. Cook for 5-7 minutes on each side until golden brown and crispy.
6. Remove the pancakes from the skillet and place them on a paper towel to remove excess oil.
7. Serve the potato pancakes warm or with a low-sodium sauce if desired.

NUTRITIONAL INFORMATION:

Calories: 180 | **Protein:** 4 g | **Carbohydrates:** 30 g | **Dietary Fiber:** 2 g | **Sugars:** 2 g | **Fat:** 5 g | **Sodium:** 50 mg | **Potassium:** 300 mg | **Phosphorus:** 70 mg

Oatmeal with Sliced Peaches

Yield: 1 serving | **Prep time:** 5 minutes | **Cook time:** 10 minutes

INGREDIENTS:

- 1/2 cup rolled oats
- 1 cup water or low-potassium milk alternative (like rice milk)
- 1 small peach, sliced
- 1 tablespoon honey or sugar (optional)
- A pinch of cinnamon

DIRECTIONS:

1. Bring water or a low-potassium milk alternative to a boil in a small saucepan.
2. Add the rolled oats and reduce the heat to a simmer.
3. Cook the oats for 5-7 minutes, stirring occasionally, until they reach your desired consistency.
4. Remove the saucepan from the heat and let the oatmeal cool slightly.
5. Stir in a pinch of cinnamon and sweeten with honey or sugar if desired.
6. Top the oatmeal with the sliced peaches.
7. Serve warm, enjoying the natural sweetness and flavor of the peaches with the oatmeal.

NUTRITIONAL INFORMATION:

Calories: 250 | **Protein:** 6 g | **Carbohydrates:** 50 g | **Dietary Fiber:** 5 g | **Sugars:** 20 g | **Fat:** 3 g | **Sodium:** 30 mg | **Potassium:** 250 mg | **Phosphorus:** 150 mg

Creamy Rice Cereal with Apples

Yield: 1 serving | **Prep time:** 5 minutes | **Cook time:** 20 minutes

INGREDIENTS:

- 1/4 cup rice (short-grain rice works best for creaminess)
- 1 cup water
- 1/2 apple, peeled and diced
- 1/4 cup low-fat milk or almond milk
- 1 tablespoon honey or sugar (optional)
- A pinch of cinnamon

DIRECTIONS:

1. Rinse the rice under cold water until the water runs clear.
2. In a small saucepan, combine the rice and water. Bring to a boil over medium heat.
3. Reduce the heat to low and simmer, covered, for about 15 minutes, or until the rice is soft and the water is mostly absorbed.
4. Add the diced apple, milk, and cinnamon to the saucepan with the rice. Stir well.
5. Continue to cook for another 5 minutes, stirring occasionally, until the mixture reaches a creamy consistency.
6. Remove from heat and sweeten with honey or sugar if desired.
7. Serve the creamy rice cereal warm, garnished with a sprinkle of cinnamon.

NUTRITIONAL INFORMATION:

Calories: 210 | **Protein:** 4 g | **Carbohydrates:** 45 g | **Dietary Fiber:** 2 g | **Sugars:** 15 g | **Fat:** 2 g | **Sodium:** 30 mg | **Potassium:** 150 mg | **Phosphorus:** 80 mg

Egg White and Tomato Scramble

Yield: 1 serving | **Prep time:** 5 minutes | **Cook time:** 5 minutes

INGREDIENTS:

- 3 egg whites
- 1 small tomato, diced
- 1 teaspoon olive oil
- A pinch of black pepper
- A pinch of garlic powder
- A few leaves of fresh basil, chopped (optional)

DIRECTIONS:

1. Heat olive oil in a non-stick skillet over medium heat.
2. Add the diced tomato to the skillet and cook for about 2 minutes until slightly softened.
3. Whisk the egg whites, black pepper, and garlic powder in a bowl.
4. Pour the egg whites over the tomatoes in the skillet.
5. Cook, stirring occasionally, until the egg whites are fully cooked and scrambled, about 3 minutes.
6. Remove from heat and sprinkle with fresh basil if using.
7. Serve the egg white and tomato scramble hot.

NUTRITIONAL INFORMATION:

Calories: 120 | **Protein:** 15 g | **Carbohydrates:** 5 g | **Dietary Fiber:** 1 g | **Sugars:** 3 g | **Fat:** 5 g | **Sodium:** 110 mg | **Potassium:** 250 mg | **Phosphorus:** 45 mg

Breakfast Rice Bowl with Mixed Veggies

Yield: 1 serving | **Prep time:** 5 minutes | **Cook time:** 15 minutes

INGREDIENTS:

- 1/2 cup cooked white rice
- 1/4 cup diced bell peppers (red or green)
- 1/4 cup diced carrots
- 1/4 cup chopped broccoli
- 1 egg
- 1 teaspoon olive oil
- A pinch of black pepper
- A pinch of garlic powder
- 1 tablespoon low-sodium soy sauce (optional)

DIRECTIONS:

1. Heat olive oil in a non-stick skillet over medium heat.
2. Add the diced bell peppers, carrots, and broccoli to the skillet. Sauté for about 5 minutes until the vegetables are tender.
3. Push the vegetables to one side of the skillet. Crack the egg into the other side and scramble it, mixing it gently with the vegetables.
4. Add the cooked rice to the skillet. Sprinkle with black pepper and garlic powder.
5. Stir everything together and cook for another 3-4 minutes until the rice is heated and the egg is fully cooked.
6. Drizzle with low-sodium soy sauce if using, and mix well.
7. Serve the rice and vegetable bowl hot.

NUTRITIONAL INFORMATION:

Calories: 300 | **Protein:** 10 g | **Carbohydrates:** 40 g | **Dietary Fiber:** 3 g | **Sugars:** 3 g | **Fat:** 10 g | **Sodium:** 200 mg (300 mg with soy sauce) | **Potassium:** 250 mg | **Phosphorus:** 150 mg

Baked Sweet Potato with Cinnamon

Yield: 1 serving | **Prep time:** 5 minutes | **Cook time:** 45 minutes

INGREDIENTS:

- 1 small sweet potato
- A pinch of cinnamon
- A drizzle of honey or maple syrup (optional)

DIRECTIONS:

1. Preheat your oven to 400°F (200°C).
2. Wash the sweet potato thoroughly and pierce it several times with a fork.
3. Place the sweet potato on a baking sheet lined with aluminum foil or parchment paper.
4. Bake in the preheated oven for about 45 minutes or until the sweet potato is tender all the way through.
5. Remove the sweet potato from the oven and let it cool slightly.
6. Split the sweet potato open and sprinkle with cinnamon.
7. Drizzle with honey or maple syrup if desired.
8. Serve warm.

NUTRITIONAL INFORMATION:

Calories: 100 | **Protein:** 2 g | **Carbohydrates:** 23 g | **Dietary Fiber:** 4 g | **Sugars:** 5 g (7 g with honey) | **Fat:** 0 g | **Sodium:** 70 mg | **Potassium:** 440 mg | **Phosphorus:** 60 mg

Kidney-Friendly Granola with Almond Milk

Yield: 1 serving | **Prep time:** 10 minutes | **Cook time:** 20 minutes

INGREDIENTS:

- 1/2 cup rolled oats
- 1 tablespoon sliced almonds
- 1 tablespoon honey or maple syrup
- 1/2 teaspoon vanilla extract
- A pinch of cinnamon
- 1/2 cup almond milk

DIRECTIONS:

1. Preheat your oven to 325°F (160°C).
2. Mix the rolled oats, sliced almonds, cinnamon, and vanilla extract in a bowl.
3. Drizzle honey or maple syrup over the oat mixture and stir until evenly coated.
4. Spread the mixture on a baking sheet lined with parchment paper.
5. Bake in the preheated oven for 15-20 minutes, stirring halfway through, until the granola is golden brown and crispy.
6. Remove the granola from the oven and let it cool completely.
7. Serve the granola with almond milk.

NUTRITIONAL INFORMATION:

Calories: 250 | **Protein:** 6 g | **Carbohydrates:** 38 g | **Dietary Fiber:** 5 g | **Sugars:** 15 g | **Fat:** 9 g | **Sodium:** 30 mg | **Potassium:** 150 mg | **Phosphorus:** 120 mg

Low-Sodium Vegetable Frittata

Yield: 1 serving | **Prep time:** 10 minutes | **Cook time:** 15 minutes

INGREDIENTS:

- 2 eggs
- 1/4 cup diced bell pepper
- 1/4 cup chopped spinach
- 1/4 cup diced tomato
- 1 tablespoon diced onion
- 1 teaspoon olive oil
- A pinch of black pepper
- 1 tablespoon grated low-sodium cheese (optional)

DIRECTIONS:

1. Preheat the oven to 375°F (190°C).

2. In a bowl, beat the eggs with black pepper until well combined.

3. Heat olive oil in an oven-safe non-stick skillet over medium heat. Add the diced bell pepper, onion, and sauté for about 3 minutes.

4. Add the chopped spinach and diced tomato to the skillet and cook for 2 minutes.

5. Pour the beaten eggs over the vegetables in the skillet, ensuring an even distribution. Cook without stirring for about 2 minutes until the edges start to set.

6. Sprinkle grated low-sodium cheese over the top if using.

7. Transfer the skillet to the preheated oven and bake for 10 minutes or until the frittata is set and lightly golden on top.

8. Remove from the oven, let it cool slightly, then slide it onto a plate and serve.

NUTRITIONAL INFORMATION:

Calories: 220 | **Protein:** 14 g | **Carbohydrates:** 8 g | **Dietary Fiber:** 2 g | **Sugars:** 4 g | **Fat:** 14 g (15 g with cheese) | **Sodium:** 180 mg | **Potassium:** 250 mg | **Phosphorus:** 180 mg

Quinoa Porridge with Mixed Berries

Yield: 1 serving | **Prep time:** 5 minutes | **Cook time:** 15 minutes

INGREDIENTS:

- 1/4 cup quinoa, rinsed
- 3/4 cup water
- 1/4 cup low-fat milk or almond milk
- 1/4 cup mixed berries (such as blueberries, raspberries, and strawberries)
- 1 tablespoon honey or maple syrup
- A pinch of cinnamon

DIRECTIONS:

1. In a small saucepan, combine rinsed quinoa and water. Bring to a boil over medium heat.

2. Reduce heat to low, cover, and simmer for about 15 minutes, or until the quinoa is cooked and the water is absorbed.

3. Stir in the milk and cook for another 2-3 minutes until the mixture is creamy.

4. Remove from heat and let it cool slightly.

5. Stir in the mixed berries, honey or maple syrup, and cinnamon.

6. Serve the quinoa porridge warm, garnished with additional berries if desired.

NUTRITIONAL INFORMATION:

Calories: 250 | **Protein:** 8 g | **Carbohydrates:** 45 g | **Dietary Fiber:** 5 g | **Sugars:** 15 g | **Fat:** 4 g | **Sodium:** 30 mg | **Potassium:** 300 mg | **Phosphorus:** 150 mg

CHAPTER 6

Lunch Recipes

Chicken and Rice Casserole
(Low Sodium)

Yield: 1 serving | **Prep time:** 10 minutes | **Cook time:** 30 minutes

INGREDIENTS:

- 4 oz boneless, skinless chicken breast, cut into small pieces
- 1/2 cup cooked white rice
- 1/4 cup low-sodium chicken broth
- 1/4 cup diced carrots
- 1/4 cup diced celery
- 1/4 cup diced onion
- 1 clove garlic, minced
- 1 teaspoon olive oil
- A pinch of black pepper
- A pinch of dried thyme
- 1 tablespoon low-sodium cheese, grated (optional)

DIRECTIONS:

1. Preheat your oven to 350°F (175°C).
2. Heat olive oil in a skillet over medium heat. Add the chicken pieces and cook until lightly browned and cooked through.
3. Remove the chicken from the skillet and set aside.
4. Add the diced carrots, celery, onion, and minced garlic in the same skillet. Sauté until the vegetables are tender.
5. Combine the cooked chicken, sautéed vegetables, cooked rice, low-sodium chicken broth, black pepper, and dried thyme in a small casserole dish.
6. Stir well to mix all the ingredients.
7. Sprinkle the top with grated low-sodium cheese if using.
8. Bake in the oven for 20 minutes or until the casserole is heated and the cheese is melted.
9. Serve hot.

NUTRITIONAL INFORMATION:

Calories: 350 | **Protein:** 28 g | **Carbohydrates:** 40 g | **Dietary Fiber:** 2 g | **Sugars:** 3 g | **Fat:** 10 g | **Sodium:** 150 mg | **Potassium:** 400 mg | **Phosphorus:** 250 mg

Renal-Friendly Chicken Wrap

Yield: 1 serving | **Prep time:** 10 minutes | **Cook time:** 10 minutes

INGREDIENTS:

- 1 boneless, skinless chicken breast (about 3 oz)
- 1 low-sodium whole wheat tortilla
- 1/4 cup shredded lettuce
- 1/4 cup diced tomato
- 2 tablespoons diced cucumber
- 1 tablespoon low-fat mayonnaise
- A pinch of black pepper
- 1 teaspoon olive oil

DIRECTIONS:

1. Season the chicken breast with black pepper. Heat olive oil in a skillet over medium heat and cook the chicken for 5 minutes on each side or until fully cooked. Let it cool slightly, then slice thinly.
2. Lay the low-sodium tortilla flat on a plate.
3. Spread the low-fat mayonnaise evenly over the tortilla.
4. Place the sliced chicken, shredded lettuce, diced tomato, and cucumber in the center of the tortilla.
5. To enclose the filling, Roll the tortilla tightly, folding in the sides as you roll.
6. Cut the wrap in half and serve.

NUTRITIONAL INFORMATION:

Calories: 350 | **Protein:** 28 g | **Carbohydrates:** 35 g | **Dietary Fiber:** 5 g | **Sugars:** 3 g | **Fat:** 12 g | **Sodium:** 320 mg | **Potassium:** 400 mg | **Phosphorus:** 220 mg

Grilled Chicken Salad with Low-Sodium Dressing

Yield: 1 serving | **Prep time:** 15 minutes | **Cook time:** 10 minutes

INGREDIENTS:

- 1 boneless, skinless chicken breast
- 2 cups mixed salad greens
- 1/4 cup sliced cucumber
- 1/4 cup cherry tomatoes, halved
- 1 tablespoon olive oil
- 1 tablespoon vinegar (apple cider or white)
- A pinch of black pepper
- A pinch of garlic powder
- A pinch of dried herbs (like oregano or basil)
- Lemon wedges (for serving)

DIRECTIONS:

1. Preheat your grill to medium-high heat.
2. Season the chicken breast with black pepper and garlic powder.
3. Grill the chicken for 5 minutes per side or until fully cooked and the internal temperature reaches 165°F (75°C).
4. Let the chicken rest briefly, then slice it thinly.
5. In a large bowl, toss the salad greens, sliced cucumber, and cherry tomatoes.
6. Whisk the olive oil, vinegar, and dried herbs in a small bowl to make the dressing.
7. Drizzle the dressing over the salad and toss gently to coat.
8. Arrange the salad on a plate and top with the grilled chicken slices.
9. Serve with lemon wedges on the side.

NUTRITIONAL INFORMATION:

Calories: 320 | **Protein:** 28 g | **Carbohydrates:** 6 g | **Dietary Fiber:** 2 g | **Sugars:** 3 g | **Fat:** 20 g | **Sodium:** 70 mg | **Potassium:** 500 mg | **Phosphorus:** 250 mg

Egg Salad with Low-Sodium Mayonnaise

Yield: 1 serving | **Prep time:** 5 minutes | **Cook time:** 10 minutes

INGREDIENTS:

- 2 eggs
- 2 tablespoons low-sodium mayonnaise
- 1 tablespoon chopped celery
- 1 tablespoon chopped red onion
- A pinch of black pepper
- A pinch of paprika (optional)

DIRECTIONS:

1. Place the eggs in a saucepan and cover with water. Bring to a boil, reduce the heat, and simmer for 10 minutes.
2. Remove the eggs from the heat, cool them under cold running water, and peel them.
3. In a bowl, chop the hard-boiled eggs and mix with low-sodium mayonnaise, celery, and red onion.
4. Add a pinch of black pepper and paprika and stir to combine.
5. Serve the egg salad alone, on a bed of lettuce, or low-sodium bread for a sandwich.

NUTRITIONAL INFORMATION:

Calories: 230 | **Protein:** 12 g | **Carbohydrates:** 2 g | **Dietary Fiber:** 0.5 g | **Sugars:** 1.5 g | **Fat:** 20 g | **Sodium:** 200 mg | **Potassium:** 140 mg | **Phosphorus:** 180 mg

Vegetable Stir-Fry with White Rice

Yield: 1 serving | **Prep time:** 10 minutes | **Cook time:** 15 minutes

INGREDIENTS:

- 1/2 cup cooked white rice
- 1/4 cup sliced bell peppers
- 1/4 cup broccoli florets
- 1/4 cup sliced carrots
- 1/4 cup snow peas
- 1 teaspoon olive oil
- 1 clove garlic, minced
- 1 tablespoon low-sodium soy sauce
- A pinch of black pepper
- A sprinkle of sesame seeds (optional)

DIRECTIONS:

1. Cook the white rice according to package instructions and set aside.
2. Heat olive oil in a skillet or wok over medium-high heat.
3. Add the garlic and stir-fry for about 30 seconds until fragrant.
4. Add the sliced bell peppers, broccoli, carrots, and snow peas to the skillet. Stir-fry for about 5 minutes until the vegetables are tender but still crisp.
5. Drizzle the low-sodium soy sauce over the vegetables and add black pepper. Stir well to combine.
6. Serve the vegetable stir-fry over the cooked white rice.
7. Garnish with sesame seeds, if desired.

NUTRITIONAL INFORMATION:

Calories: 220 | **Protein:** 5 g | **Carbohydrates:** 35 g | **Dietary Fiber:** 3 g | **Sugars:** 5 g | **Fat:** 7 g | **Sodium:** 150 mg | **Potassium:** 300 mg | **Phosphorus:** 100 mg

Low-Potassium Tomato Soup

Yield: 1 serving | **Prep time:** 5 minutes | **Cook time:** 20 minutes

INGREDIENTS:

- 1 cup low-potassium canned tomatoes (crushed or pureed)
- 1/4 cup diced onion
- 1 clove garlic, minced
- 1 cup low-sodium vegetable broth
- 1 teaspoon olive oil
- A pinch of black pepper
- A pinch of dried basil
- A pinch of dried oregano
- 1 tablespoon low-fat milk or cream (optional)

DIRECTIONS:

1. Heat olive oil in a saucepan over medium heat. Add the diced onion and minced garlic, sautéing until the onion is translucent, about 3-4 minutes.
2. Add the low-potassium canned tomatoes, low-sodium vegetable broth, black pepper, dried basil, and dried oregano to the saucepan. Stir to combine.
3. Bring the mixture to a boil, then reduce the heat to low and simmer for 15 minutes, allowing the flavors to meld together.
4. Add low-fat milk or cream for a creamier texture and stir well if desired.
5. Remove from heat and use an immersion blender to blend the soup until smooth (optional step).
6. Serve the tomato soup hot.

NUTRITIONAL INFORMATION:

Calories: 120 | **Protein:** 3 g | **Carbohydrates:** 18 g | **Dietary Fiber:** 3 g | **Sugars:** 10 g | **Fat:** 5 g | **Sodium:** 200 mg | **Potassium:** 300 mg | **Phosphorus:** 50 mg

Zucchini Noodles with Tomato Sauce

Yield: 1 serving | **Prep time:** 10 minutes | **Cook time:** 15 minutes

INGREDIENTS:

- 1 medium zucchini
- 1/2 cup low-sodium canned tomato sauce
- 1 clove garlic, minced
- 1 teaspoon olive oil
- A pinch of dried oregano
- A pinch of dried basil
- Black pepper to taste
- Grated Parmesan cheese for garnish (optional)

DIRECTIONS:

1. Use a spiralizer or a vegetable peeler to make noodles from the zucchini. Set aside.
2. In a skillet, heat the olive oil over medium heat. Add the minced garlic and sauté for about 1 minute.
3. Add the low-sodium tomato sauce to the skillet and season it with dried oregano, basil, and black pepper. Simmer for about 10 minutes, stirring occasionally.
4. Add the zucchini noodles to the skillet with the tomato sauce. Toss gently and cook for 2-3 minutes until the noodles are tender but firm.
5. Remove from heat and transfer to a serving plate.
6. Sprinkle with grated Parmesan cheese if desired.
7. Serve immediately.

NUTRITIONAL INFORMATION:

Calories: 150 | **Protein:** 4 g | **Carbohydrates:** 18 g | **Dietary Fiber:** 4 g | **Sugars:** 8 g | **Fat:** 8 g | **Sodium:** 200 mg | **Potassium:** 500 mg | **Phosphorus:** 100 mg

Baked Lemon Pepper Cod

Yield: 1 serving | **Prep time:** 5 minutes | **Cook time:** 12 minutes

INGREDIENTS:

- 1 cod fillet (about 6 oz)
- Juice of 1/2 lemon
- A pinch of black pepper
- A pinch of garlic powder
- 1 teaspoon olive oil
- Fresh parsley for garnish (optional)

DIRECTIONS:

1. Preheat your oven to 400°F (200°C).
2. Place the cod fillet on a baking sheet lined with parchment paper or lightly greased with olive oil.
3. Drizzle lemon juice over the cod. Season with black pepper and garlic powder.
4. Drizzle the top of the fillet with olive oil.
5. Bake in the oven for about 12 minutes or until the fish flakes easily with a fork.
6. Remove from the oven and garnish with fresh parsley, if desired.
7. Serve hot.

NUTRITIONAL INFORMATION:

Calories: 200 | **Protein:** 35 g | **Carbohydrates:** 1 g | **Dietary Fiber:** 0 g | **Sugars:** 0 g | **Fat:** 6 g | **Sodium:** 100 mg | **Potassium:** 500 mg | **Phosphorus:** 300 mg

Low-Phosphorus Pasta Primavera

Yield: 1 serving | **Prep time:** 10 minutes | **Cook time:** 15 minutes

INGREDIENTS:

- 1 cup cooked low-phosphorus pasta (e.g., white or rice pasta)
- 1/4 cup sliced zucchini
- 1/4 cup sliced bell pepper
- 1/4 cup cherry tomatoes, halved
- 1 tablespoon olive oil
- 1 clove garlic, minced
- 1/4 cup low-sodium vegetable broth
- A pinch of black pepper
- A pinch of dried Italian herbs
- 1 tablespoon grated Parmesan cheese (optional)

DIRECTIONS:

1. Cook the pasta according to package instructions. Drain and set aside.
2. Heat olive oil in a skillet over medium heat. Add garlic and sauté for about 1 minute.
3. Add zucchini and bell pepper to the skillet. Cook for about 3 minutes, until slightly softened.
4. Add cherry tomatoes and cook for another 2 minutes.
5. Pour in the low-sodium vegetable broth and bring to a simmer. Season with black pepper and Italian herbs.
6. Add the cooked pasta to the skillet. Toss everything together and heat through for 2-3 minutes.
7. Serve the pasta primavera in a bowl. Sprinkle with grated Parmesan cheese, if desired.

NUTRITIONAL INFORMATION:

Calories: 350 | **Protein:** 8 g | **Carbohydrates:** 45 g | **Dietary Fiber:** 3 g | **Sugars:** 4 g | **Fat:** 16 g | **Sodium:** 150 mg | **Potassium:** 300 mg | **Phosphorus:** 100 mg

Kidney-Friendly Turkey Burger

Yield: 1 serving | **Prep time:** 10 minutes | **Cook time:** 10 minutes

INGREDIENTS:

- 4 oz ground turkey (lean)
- 1 tablespoon diced onion
- A pinch of black pepper
- 1 teaspoon olive oil
- 1 low-sodium whole wheat bun
- Lettuce leaves
- 1 slice of tomato
- 1 tablespoon low-sodium ketchup or mustard (optional)

DIRECTIONS:

1. Mix the ground turkey, diced onion, and black pepper in a bowl.
2. Form the mixture into a patty.
3. Heat olive oil in a skillet over medium heat.
4. Cook the turkey patty for 5 minutes on each side until fully cooked and the internal temperature reaches 165°F (74°C).
5. Toast the low-sodium bun lightly, if desired.
6. Place the cooked turkey burger on the bun.
7. Top with lettuce, tomato, and low-sodium ketchup or mustard if using.
8. Serve the turkey burger immediately.

NUTRITIONAL INFORMATION:

Calories: 320 | **Protein:** 28 g | **Carbohydrates:** 28 g | **Dietary Fiber:** 3 g | **Sugars:** 5 g | **Fat:** 12 g | **Sodium:** 200 mg | **Potassium:** 300 mg | **Phosphorus:** 250 mg

Beef Stew with Low-Potassium Vegetables

Yield: 1 serving | **Prep time:** 15 minutes | **Cook time:** 60 minutes

INGREDIENTS:

- 4 oz beef stew meat, cut into cubes
- 1/2 cup sliced carrots
- 1/2 cup chopped green beans
- 1/4 cup diced celery
- 1/4 cup diced onion
- 1 clove garlic, minced
- 1 cup low-sodium beef broth
- 1 teaspoon olive oil
- A pinch of black pepper
- A pinch of dried thyme
- 1 bay leaf

DIRECTIONS:

1. Heat olive oil in a pot over medium heat. Add beef cubes and cook until browned on all sides.
2. Remove the beef and set aside. Add onion, garlic, carrots, green beans, and celery in the same pot. Sauté for about 5 minutes.
3. Return the beef to the pot. Add low-sodium beef broth, black pepper, dried thyme, and a bay leaf.
4. Bring to a boil, then reduce heat to low, cover, and simmer for about 1 hour, or until the beef is tender and the vegetables are cooked.
5. Remove the bay leaf before serving.
6. Serve the beef stew hot.

NUTRITIONAL INFORMATION:

Calories: 350 | **Protein:** 35 g | **Carbohydrates:** 15 g | **Dietary Fiber:** 3 g | **Sugars:** 5 g | **Fat:** 15 g | **Sodium:** 200 mg | **Potassium:** 450 mg | **Phosphorus:** 300 mg

Cauliflower Rice and Vegetable Medley

Yield: 1 serving | **Prep time:** 10 minutes | **Cook time:** 15 minutes

INGREDIENTS:

- 1 cup riced cauliflower (fresh or frozen)
- 1/4 cup diced carrots
- 1/4 cup chopped green beans
- 1/4 cup diced bell peppers
- 1 tablespoon olive oil
- 1 clove garlic, minced
- A pinch of black pepper
- A pinch of dried herbs (such as thyme or parsley)
- 1 tablespoon low-sodium soy sauce (optional)

DIRECTIONS:

1. Heat olive oil in a skillet over medium heat. Add minced garlic and sauté for about 1 minute until fragrant.

2. Add the diced carrots, chopped green beans, and bell peppers to the skillet. Stir-fry for about 5 minutes until the vegetables start to soften.

3. Stir in the riced cauliflower, black pepper, and dried herbs. Cook for another 5-7 minutes, stirring occasionally, until the cauliflower is tender.

4. If using, drizzle low-sodium soy sauce over the mixture and stir well to combine.

5. Remove from heat once everything is heated and the vegetables are cooked to your liking.

6. Serve the cauliflower rice and vegetable medley hot.

NUTRITIONAL INFORMATION:

Calories: 180 | **Protein:** 4 g | **Carbohydrates:** 18 g | **Dietary Fiber:** 5 g | **Sugars:** 6 g | **Fat:** 10 g | **Sodium:** 150 mg (200 mg with soy sauce) | **Potassium:** 400 mg | **Phosphorus:** 100 mg

Grilled Shrimp with Garlic and Herbs

Yield: 1 serving | **Prep time:** 10 minutes | **Cook time:** 6 minutes

INGREDIENTS:

- 6 large shrimp, peeled and deveined
- 1 clove garlic, minced
- 1 tablespoon olive oil
- A pinch of black pepper
- A pinch of dried parsley
- A pinch of dried basil
- Lemon wedges for serving

DIRECTIONS:

1. Combine the minced garlic, olive oil, black pepper, parsley, and basil in a small bowl. Mix well to create a marinade.

2. Add the shrimp to the marinade, ensuring they are well coated. Let them marinate for about 10 minutes.

3. Preheat your grill or grill pan to medium-high heat.

4. Place the marinated shrimp on the grill. Cook for about 3 minutes on each side or until the shrimp are pink and opaque.

5. Remove the shrimp from the grill and serve with lemon wedges on the side.

NUTRITIONAL INFORMATION:

Calories: 180 | **Protein:** 18 g | **Carbohydrates:** 2 g | **Dietary Fiber:** 0 g | **Sugars:** 0 g | **Fat:** 11 g | **Sodium:** 150 mg | **Potassium:** 200 mg | **Phosphorus:** 180 mg

Lentil Soup

(Low Potassium Recipe)

Yield: 1 serving | **Prep time:** 10 minutes | **Cook time:** 30 minutes

INGREDIENTS:

- 1/4 cup dried lentils, rinsed
- 1 cup low-sodium vegetable broth
- 1/4 cup diced carrots
- 1/4 cup diced celery
- 1 tablespoon diced onion
- 1 clove garlic, minced
- 1 teaspoon olive oil
- A pinch of black pepper
- A pinch of dried thyme
- 1 bay leaf

DIRECTIONS:

1. In a saucepan, heat the olive oil over medium heat. Add the diced onion and garlic, and sauté until the onion is translucent.
2. Add the diced carrots and celery to the saucepan. Cook for about 5 minutes, stirring occasionally.
3. Add the rinsed lentils, low-sodium vegetable broth, black pepper, dried thyme, and bay leaf to the saucepan. Stir to combine.
4. Bring the mixture to a boil, then reduce heat to low, cover, and simmer for about 25 minutes or until the lentils are tender.
5. Remove the bay leaf before serving.
6. Serve the lentil soup hot.

NUTRITIONAL INFORMATION:

Calories: 200 | **Protein:** 12 g | **Carbohydrates:** 30 g | **Dietary Fiber:** 8 g | **Sugars:** 4 g | **Fat:** 4 g | **Sodium:** 150 mg | **Potassium:** 350 mg | **Phosphorus:** 150 mg

Rice and Beans with Low-Sodium Seasoning

Yield: 1 serving | **Prep time:** 10 minutes | **Cook time:** 20 minutes

INGREDIENTS:

- 1/2 cup cooked white rice
- 1/2 cup canned low-sodium black beans drained and rinsed
- 1 tablespoon olive oil
- 1/4 cup diced bell pepper
- 1/4 cup diced onion
- 1 clove garlic, minced
- A pinch of black pepper
- A pinch of cumin
- A pinch of paprika
- Fresh cilantro for garnish (optional)

DIRECTIONS:

1. Heat olive oil in a skillet over medium heat. Add the diced onion, bell pepper, and sauté until softened, about 5 minutes.
2. Add the minced garlic, black pepper, cumin, and paprika to the skillet. Cook for an additional 1-2 minutes, stirring frequently.
3. Stir in the cooked rice and rinse the black beans. Cook for 5-7 minutes, stirring occasionally, until the mixture is heated.
4. Taste and adjust the seasoning if necessary.
5. Remove from heat and transfer to a serving dish.
6. Garnish with fresh cilantro if desired.
7. Serve hot as a wholesome and kidney-friendly meal.

NUTRITIONAL INFORMATION:

Calories: 350 | **Protein:** 10 g | **Carbohydrates:** 50 g | **Dietary Fiber:** 8 g | **Sugars:** 3 g | **Fat:** 12 g | **Sodium:** 150 mg | **Potassium:** 400 mg | **Phosphorus:** 150 mg

Baked Sweet Potato with Cinnamon

(small portion)

Yield: 1 serving | **Prep time:** 5 minutes | **Cook time:** 45 minutes

INGREDIENTS:

- 1 small sweet potato
- A pinch of cinnamon
- A drizzle of honey or maple syrup (optional)

DIRECTIONS:

1. Preheat your oven to 400°F (200°C).
2. Wash the sweet potato thoroughly and pierce it several times with a fork.
3. Place the sweet potato on a baking sheet lined with aluminum foil or parchment paper.
4. Bake in the preheated oven for about 45 minutes or until the sweet potato is tender all the way through.
5. Remove the sweet potato from the oven and let it cool slightly.
6. Split the sweet potato open and sprinkle with cinnamon.
7. Drizzle with honey or maple syrup if desired.
8. Serve warm.

NUTRITIONAL INFORMATION:

Calories: 100 | **Protein:** 2 g | **Carbohydrates:** 23 g | **Dietary Fiber:** 4 g | **Sugars:** 5 g (7 g with honey) | **Fat:** 0 g | **Sodium:** 70 mg | **Potassium:** 440 mg | **Phosphorus:** 60 mg

Broiled White Fish with Herbs

Yield: 1 serving | **Prep time:** 5 minutes | **Cook time:** 10 minutes

INGREDIENTS:

- 1 white fish fillet (such as cod or tilapia, about 6 oz)
- 1 teaspoon olive oil
- A pinch of dried thyme
- A pinch of dried parsley
- A pinch of black pepper
- Lemon wedges for serving

DIRECTIONS:

1. Preheat your broiler high and position a rack about 6 inches from the heat source.
2. Lightly brush both sides of the fish fillet with olive oil.
3. Sprinkle the thyme, parsley, and black pepper evenly over the fish.
4. Place the seasoned fish on a broiler pan or a baking sheet lined with foil.
5. Broil for 5 minutes; carefully flip the fish over, and broil for 3-5 minutes or until the fish flakes easily with a fork.
6. Remove the fish from the oven and serve hot with lemon wedges on the side.

NUTRITIONAL INFORMATION:

Calories: 200 | **Protein:** 35 g | **Carbohydrates:** 0 g | **Dietary Fiber:** 0 g | **Sugars:** 0 g | **Fat:** 5 g | **Sodium:** 100 mg | **Potassium:** 450 mg | **Phosphorus:** 250 mg

Tuna Salad Sandwich on Low-Sodium Bread

Yield: 1 serving | **Prep time:** 10 minutes | **Cook time:** 0 minutes

INGREDIENTS:

- 1 can (3 oz) low-sodium tuna, drained
- 2 tablespoons low-fat mayonnaise
- 1 tablespoon diced celery
- 1 tablespoon diced red onion
- A pinch of black pepper
- 2 slices low-sodium bread
- Lettuce leaves (optional)
- Thinly sliced cucumber (optional)

DIRECTIONS:

1. Mix the drained tuna, low-fat mayonnaise, diced celery, and red onion in a small bowl. Add a pinch of black pepper to taste.

2. Spread the tuna mixture evenly on one slice of low-sodium bread.

3. Add lettuce leaves and thinly sliced cucumber to the tuna mixture for added crunch and flavor.

4. Cover with the other slice of bread.

5. Cut the sandwich in half, if preferred.

6. Serve immediately for a fresh and satisfying meal.

NUTRITIONAL INFORMATION:

Calories: 280 | **Protein:** 25 g | **Carbohydrates:** 28 g | **Dietary Fiber:** 4 g | **Sugars:** 4 g | **Fat:** 9 g | **Sodium:** 300 mg | **Potassium:** 200 mg | **Phosphorus:** 250 mg

Quinoa Salad with Lemon Vinaigrette

Yield: 1 serving | **Prep time:** 10 minutes | **Cook time:** 15 minutes

INGREDIENTS:

- 1/4 cup quinoa
- 1/2 cup water
- 1/4 cup diced cucumber
- 1/4 cup cherry tomatoes, halved
- 1 tablespoon chopped red onion
- 1 tablespoon olive oil
- Juice of 1/2 lemon
- A pinch of black pepper
- A pinch of dried parsley

DIRECTIONS:

1. Rinse quinoa under cold water. In a small saucepan, bring water to a boil. Add quinoa, reduce heat to low, cover, and simmer for about 15 minutes or until all water is absorbed.

2. Remove the quinoa from the heat and let it cool to room temperature.

3. Combine cooled quinoa, diced cucumber, cherry tomatoes, and chopped red onion in a salad bowl.

4. Whisk olive oil, lemon juice, black pepper, and dried parsley in a small bowl to create the vinaigrette.

5. Drizzle the vinaigrette over the salad and toss to coat evenly.

6. Serve the quinoa salad chilled or at room temperature.

NUTRITIONAL INFORMATION:

Calories: 280 | **Protein:** 6 g | **Carbohydrates:** 35 g | **Dietary Fiber:** 4 g | **Sugars:** 2 g | **Fat:** 14 g | **Sodium:** 10 mg | **Potassium:** 250 mg | **Phosphorus:** 150 mg

Cabbage and Carrot Slaw

Yield: 1 serving | **Prep time:** 15 minutes | **Cook time:** 0 minutes

INGREDIENTS:

- 1 cup shredded green cabbage
- 1/2 cup shredded carrots
- 1 tablespoon apple cider vinegar
- 1 teaspoon honey
- 1 tablespoon olive oil
- A pinch of black pepper
- A pinch of salt (optional)

DIRECTIONS:

1. Combine the shredded green cabbage and carrots in a large bowl.
2. Whisk the apple cider vinegar, honey, and olive oil in a small bowl to create the dressing.
3. Pour the dressing over the cabbage and carrot mixture.
4. Season with black pepper and a pinch of salt if desired.
5. Toss the slaw until it is evenly coated with the dressing.
6. Let the slaw sit for about 10 minutes to allow the flavors to meld.
7. Serve as a fresh and crunchy side dish.

NUTRITIONAL INFORMATION:

Calories: 150 | **Protein:** 2 g | **Carbohydrates:** 15 g | **Dietary Fiber:** 3 g | **Sugars:** 10 g | **Fat:** 10 g | **Sodium:** 50 mg (without added salt) | **Potassium:** 250 mg | **Phosphorus:** 40 mg

Veggie Omelette with Low-Phosphorus Cheese

Yield: 1 serving | **Prep time:** 10 minutes | **Cook time:** 5 minutes

INGREDIENTS:

- 2 eggs
- 1/4 cup diced bell peppers
- 1/4 cup diced tomatoes
- 1/4 cup chopped spinach
- 1 tablespoon diced onion
- 1 tablespoon olive oil
- 1/4 cup shredded low-phosphorus cheese (such as Swiss or mozzarella)
- A pinch of black pepper
- A pinch of garlic powder

DIRECTIONS:

1. In a bowl, beat the eggs with black pepper and garlic powder until well combined.
2. Heat olive oil in a non-stick skillet over medium heat. Add the diced onion, bell peppers, and tomatoes. Sauté for about 2 minutes until the vegetables are slightly softened.
3. Add the chopped spinach to the skillet and cook for another minute.
4. Pour the beaten eggs over the vegetables in the skillet. Tilt the skillet to ensure the eggs are evenly distributed.
5. Sprinkle the shredded low-phosphorus cheese over the egg mixture.
6. Cook the omelet for 2-3 minutes, then carefully fold it in half and cook for another minute.
7. Slide the omelet onto a plate and serve hot.

NUTRITIONAL INFORMATION:

Calories: 320 | **Protein:** 20 g | **Carbohydrates:** 6 g | **Dietary Fiber:** 1 g | **Sugars:** 3 g | **Fat:** 24 g | **Sodium:** 220 mg | **Potassium:** 300 mg | **Phosphorus:** 150 mg

Turkey and Avocado Sandwich on Low-Sodium Bread

Yield: 1 serving | **Prep time:** 5 minutes | **Cook time:** 0 minutes

INGREDIENTS:

- 2 slices of low-sodium whole-wheat bread
- 3 oz thinly sliced turkey breast (low-sodium)
- 1/4 ripe avocado, sliced
- 1 lettuce leaf
- 2 tomato slices
- 1 teaspoon mustard (optional)
- 1 teaspoon mayonnaise (low-fat, optional)

DIRECTIONS:

1. Lay the slices of low-sodium bread on a plate.
2. Spread mustard and mayonnaise on one slice of bread if using.
3. Place the lettuce leaf on the bottom slice of bread.
4. Add the sliced turkey breast on top of the lettuce.
5. Arrange the avocado slices and tomato slices over the turkey.
6. Top with the second slice of bread.
7. If preferred, Cut the sandwich in half and serve immediately.

NUTRITIONAL INFORMATION:

Calories: 350 | **Protein:** 25 g | **Carbohydrates:** 35 g | **Dietary Fiber:** 6 g | **Sugars:** 5 g | **Fat:** 12 g | **Sodium:** 250 mg | **Potassium:** 500 mg | **Phosphorus:** 200 mg

Pasta with Olive Oil and Garlic
(Low Phosphorus)

Yield: 1 serving | **Prep time:** 5 minutes | **Cook time:** 10 minutes

INGREDIENTS:

- 1 cup cooked low-phosphorus pasta (such as white or rice pasta)
- 2 tablespoons olive oil
- 2 cloves garlic, minced
- A pinch of black pepper
- A pinch of dried parsley or basil
- Grated Parmesan cheese for garnish (optional, and use a low-phosphorus variety if available)

DIRECTIONS:

1. Cook the pasta according to package instructions until al dente. Drain and set aside.
2. In a skillet, heat olive oil over medium heat.
3. Add minced garlic to the skillet and sauté for about 1-2 minutes, until fragrant but not browned.
4. Add the cooked pasta to the skillet with the olive oil and garlic. Toss to coat the pasta evenly.
5. Season with black pepper and dried parsley or basil.
6. Transfer the pasta to a serving dish.
7. If desired, sprinkle with a small amount of grated Parmesan cheese.
8. Serve the pasta warm.

NUTRITIONAL INFORMATION:

Calories: 400 | **Protein:** 8 g | **Carbohydrates:** 42 g | **Dietary Fiber:** 2 g | **Sugars:** 2 g | **Fat:** 22 g | **Sodium:** 30 mg | **Potassium:** 100 mg | **Phosphorus:** 100 mg

Pan-seared tilapia with Lemon

Yield: 1 serving | **Prep time:** 5 minutes | **Cook time:** 8 minutes

INGREDIENTS:

- 1 tilapia fillet (about 6 oz)
- 1 teaspoon olive oil
- Juice of 1/2 lemon
- A pinch of black pepper
- A pinch of dried parsley
- Lemon slices for garnish

DIRECTIONS:

1. Pat the tilapia fillet dry with paper towels.
2. Season both sides of the fillet with black pepper and dried parsley.
3. Heat olive oil in a non-stick skillet over medium-high heat.
4. Place the tilapia fillet in the skillet once the oil is hot.
5. Cook for about 4 minutes on one side, then flip and cook for 3-4 minutes on the other side or until the fish flakes easily with a fork.
6. Squeeze the lemon juice evenly over the cooked fillet.
7. Serve the tilapia garnished with lemon slices.

NUTRITIONAL INFORMATION:

Calories: 200 | **Protein:** 35 g | **Carbohydrates:** 1 g | **Dietary Fiber:** 0 g | **Sugars:** 0 g | **Fat:** 6 g | **Sodium:** 70 mg | **Potassium:** 450 mg | **Phosphorus:** 250 mg

Spinach and Mushroom Quiche
(Egg Whites)

Yield: 1 serving | **Prep time:** 10 minutes | **Cook time:** 25 minutes

INGREDIENTS:

- 3 egg whites
- 1/4 cup chopped fresh spinach
- 1/4 cup diced mushrooms
- 1 tablespoon diced onion
- 1 teaspoon olive oil
- 1/4 cup low-fat milk or almond milk
- A pinch of black pepper
- A pinch of garlic powder
- 2 tablespoons shredded low-phosphorus cheese (like Swiss or mozzarella)

DIRECTIONS:

1. Preheat your oven to 350°F (175°C).
2. Heat olive oil in a skillet over medium heat. Add onions and mushrooms, and sauté until softened, about 3-4 minutes.
3. Add the chopped spinach to the skillet and cook until wilted, about 1-2 minutes. Remove from heat.
4. Whisk the egg whites, low-fat milk, black pepper, and garlic powder in a bowl.
5. Stir the sautéed vegetables into the egg mixture.
6. Pour the mixture into a small, greased baking dish or pie pan. Sprinkle with shredded cheese.
7. Bake in the oven for 20 minutes or until the quiche is set and lightly golden.
8. Remove from the oven and let it cool for a few minutes before serving.

NUTRITIONAL INFORMATION:

Calories: 180 | **Protein:** 18 g | **Carbohydrates:** 6 g | **Dietary Fiber:** 1 g | **Sugars:** 3 g | **Fat:** 8 g | **Sodium:** 200 mg | **Potassium:** 300 mg | **Phosphorus:** 150 mg

Barley Soup with Carrots and Celery

Yield: 1 serving | **Prep time:** 10 minutes | **Cook time:** 30 minutes

INGREDIENTS:

- 1/4 cup pearl barley
- 1 cup low-sodium vegetable broth
- 1/4 cup diced carrots
- 1/4 cup diced celery
- 1 tablespoon diced onion
- 1 clove garlic, minced
- 1 teaspoon olive oil
- A pinch of black pepper
- A pinch of dried thyme

DIRECTIONS:

1. Rinse the barley under cold water.

2. In a saucepan, heat olive oil over medium heat. Add onion and garlic, and sauté for about 2 minutes until the onion is translucent.

3. Add diced carrots and celery to the saucepan and continue to sauté for another 3 minutes.

4. Add the rinsed barley and the low-sodium vegetable broth to the saucepan.

5. Bring the mixture to a boil, then reduce the heat to low, cover, and simmer for about 25 minutes or until the barley is tender.

6. Season the soup with black pepper and dried thyme.

7. Serve the barley soup hot.

NUTRITIONAL INFORMATION:

Calories: 220 | **Protein:** 6 g | **Carbohydrates:** 40 g | **Dietary Fiber:** 9 g | **Sugars:** 3 g | **Fat:** 4 g | **Sodium:** 150 mg | **Potassium:** 300 mg | **Phosphorus:** 100 mg

Greek Salad with Feta

(Low Sodium)

Yield: 1 serving | **Prep time:** 10 minutes | **Cook time:** 0 minutes

INGREDIENTS:

- 1 cup chopped romaine lettuce
- 1/4 cup sliced cucumber
- 1/4 cup cherry tomatoes, halved
- 1/4 cup sliced red onion
- 2 tablespoons crumbled low-sodium feta cheese
- 5 Kalamata olives, pitted
- 1 tablespoon olive oil
- 1 tablespoon red wine vinegar
- A pinch of dried oregano
- Black pepper to taste

DIRECTIONS:

1. Combine the chopped romaine lettuce, sliced cucumber, cherry tomatoes, and red onion in a salad bowl.

2. Sprinkle the crumbled low-sodium feta cheese and Kalamata olives over the salad.

3. In a small bowl, whisk together the olive oil, red wine vinegar, dried oregano, and black pepper to create the dressing.

4. Drizzle the dressing over the salad and toss gently to coat all ingredients evenly.

5. Serve the Greek salad immediately, garnished with extra-dried oregano if desired.

NUTRITIONAL INFORMATION:

Calories: 250 | **Protein:** 6 g | **Carbohydrates:** 12 g | **Dietary Fiber:** 3 g | **Sugars:** 5 g | **Fat:** 20 g | **Sodium:** 300 mg | **Potassium:** 350 mg | **Phosphorus:** 100 mg

Vegetable and Barley Stew

Yield: 1 serving | **Prep time:** 10 minutes | **Cook time:** 30 minutes

INGREDIENTS:

- 1/4 cup pearl barley
- 1 cup low-sodium vegetable broth
- 1/4 cup diced carrots
- 1/4 cup diced celery
- 1/4 cup chopped onion
- 1/4 cup diced potato
- 1 clove garlic, minced
- 1 teaspoon olive oil
- A pinch of dried thyme
- A pinch of black pepper

DIRECTIONS:

1. Rinse the barley under cold water.

2. In a saucepan, heat olive oil over medium heat. Add the onion and garlic, and sauté until the onion is translucent.

3. Add the carrots, celery, and potato to the saucepan. Cook for about 5 minutes, stirring occasionally.

4. Add the rinsed barley and low-sodium vegetable broth to the saucepan. Stir in the dried thyme and black pepper.

5. Bring the stew to a boil, then reduce the heat to low, cover, and simmer for about 25 minutes or until the barley and vegetables are tender.

6. Check the seasoning and adjust if necessary.

7. Serve the vegetable and barley stew hot.

NUTRITIONAL INFORMATION:

Calories: 250 | **Protein:** 6 g | **Carbohydrates:** 45 g | **Dietary Fiber:** 9 g | **Sugars:** 5 g | **Fat:** 5 g | **Sodium:** 150 mg | **Potassium:** 400 mg | **Phosphorus:** 100 mg

Couscous Salad with Roasted Vegetables

Yield: 1 serving | **Prep time:** 15 minutes | **Cook time:** 25 minutes

INGREDIENTS:

- 1/2 cup couscous
- 1 cup water
- 1/4 cup diced zucchini
- 1/4 cup diced bell pepper
- 1/4 cup cherry tomatoes, halved
- 1 tablespoon olive oil
- A pinch of black pepper
- A pinch of dried herbs (like thyme or basil)
- 1 tablespoon lemon juice
- 1 teaspoon balsamic vinegar
- 1 tablespoon chopped fresh parsley (optional)

DIRECTIONS:

1. Preheat your oven to 400°F (200°C).

2. Toss zucchini, bell pepper, and cherry tomatoes with olive oil, black pepper, and dried herbs.

3. Spread the vegetables on a baking sheet and roast in the oven for about 20 minutes until tender and slightly caramelized.

4. Meanwhile, bring water to a boil in a pot. Add couscous, stir, then cover and remove from heat. Let it sit for 5 minutes, then fluff it with a fork.

5. Mix the cooked couscous with roasted vegetables, lemon juice, and balsamic vinegar in a bowl.

6. Garnish with chopped fresh parsley if desired.

7. Serve the couscous salad warm or at room temperature.

NUTRITIONAL INFORMATION:

Calories: 350 | **Protein:** 8 g | **Carbohydrates:** 55 g | **Dietary Fiber:** 4 g | **Sugars:** 5 g | **Fat:** 12 g | **Sodium:** 30 mg | **Potassium:** 300 mg | **Phosphorus:** 100 mg

Ratatouille with Eggplant and Zucchini

Yield: 1 serving | **Prep time:** 15 minutes | **Cook time:** 30 minutes

INGREDIENTS:

- 1/2 small eggplant, diced
- 1 small zucchini, sliced
- 1/4 cup diced bell pepper
- 1/4 cup diced onion
- 1/2 cup canned low-sodium diced tomatoes
- 1 clove garlic, minced
- 1 teaspoon olive oil
- A pinch of dried basil
- A pinch of dried thyme
- A pinch of black pepper

DIRECTIONS:

1. Preheat your oven to 375°F (190°C).
2. In a skillet, heat olive oil over medium heat. Sauté onion and garlic until translucent.
3. Add the diced eggplant and cook for about 5 minutes, stirring occasionally.
4. Add the zucchini and bell pepper to the skillet. Continue cooking for another 5 minutes.
5. Stir in the diced tomatoes, basil, thyme, and black pepper.
6. Transfer the vegetable mixture to a baking dish.
7. Bake in the oven for 20 minutes or until the vegetables are tender.
8. Serve the ratatouille warm.

NUTRITIONAL INFORMATION:

Calories: 150 | **Protein:** 4 g | **Carbohydrates:** 20 g | **Dietary Fiber:** 7 g | **Sugars:** 10 g | **Fat:** 7 g | **Sodium:** 100 mg | **Potassium:** 500 mg | **Phosphorus:** 100 mg

Roasted Chicken Breast with Herbs

Yield: 1 serving | **Prep time:** 5 minutes | **Cook time:** 25 minutes

INGREDIENTS:

- 1 boneless, skinless chicken breast (about 6 oz)
- 1 teaspoon olive oil
- A pinch of dried rosemary
- A pinch of dried thyme
- A pinch of black pepper
- A pinch of garlic powder
- Lemon wedges for serving

DIRECTIONS:

1. Preheat your oven to 375°F (190°C).
2. Pat the chicken breast dry with paper towels.
3. Rub the chicken breast with olive oil.
4. Sprinkle the dried rosemary, thyme, black pepper, and garlic powder evenly over the chicken.
5. Place the seasoned chicken breast on a baking tray lined with parchment paper.
6. Roast in the preheated oven for about 25 minutes, or until the chicken is cooked and the internal temperature reaches 165°F (75°C).
7. Remove the chicken from the oven and let it rest for a few minutes.
8. Serve the roasted chicken breast with lemon wedges on the side.

NUTRITIONAL INFORMATION:

Calories: 220 | **Protein:** 35 g | **Carbohydrates:** 0 g | **Dietary Fiber:** 0 g | **Sugars:** 0 g | **Fat:** 8 g | **Sodium:** 70 mg | **Potassium:** 400 mg | **Phosphorus:** 250 mg

Sautéed Shrimp with Bell Peppers

Yield: 1 serving | **Prep time:** 10 minutes | **Cook time:** 10 minutes

INGREDIENTS:

- 6 large shrimp, peeled and deveined
- 1/2 cup sliced bell peppers (mix of colors)
- 1 tablespoon olive oil
- 1 clove garlic, minced
- A pinch of black pepper
- A pinch of dried oregano
- Lemon wedges for serving

DIRECTIONS:

1. Heat olive oil in a skillet over medium heat.
2. Add minced garlic to the skillet and sauté for about 1 minute until fragrant.
3. Add the sliced bell peppers to the skillet and sauté for 3 minutes until they soften.
4. Add the shrimp to the skillet with the bell peppers. Season with black pepper and dried oregano.
5. Sauté the shrimp for about 2 minutes on each side until they turn pink and are cooked through.
6. Remove from heat. Serve the shrimp and bell peppers hot with lemon wedges on the side.

NUTRITIONAL INFORMATION:

Calories: 200 | **Protein:** 18 g | **Carbohydrates:** 6 g | **Dietary Fiber:** 2 g | **Sugars:** 3 g | **Fat:** 12 g | **Sodium:** 150 mg | **Potassium:** 250 mg | **Phosphorus:** 180 mg

Beef Stir-Fry with Low-Sodium Soy Sauce

Yield: 1 serving | **Prep time:** 10 minutes | **Cook time:** 10 minutes

INGREDIENTS:

- 4 oz beef sirloin, thinly sliced
- 1/2 cup sliced bell peppers
- 1/4 cup sliced onion
- 1/4 cup broccoli florets
- 1 tablespoon olive oil
- 1 clove garlic, minced
- 1 tablespoon low-sodium soy sauce
- A pinch of black pepper
- A pinch of ginger powder

DIRECTIONS:

1. Heat olive oil in a wok or large skillet over medium-high heat.
2. Add the minced garlic and ginger powder, and stir-fry for about 30 seconds.
3. Add the thinly sliced beef to the wok and stir-fry for about 2 minutes or until it browns.
4. Add the sliced bell peppers, onion, and broccoli florets. Continue to stir-fry for another 5 minutes or until the vegetables are tender and the beef is cooked.
5. Drizzle the low-sodium soy sauce over the stir-fry and toss to combine everything well—season with black pepper.
6. Cook for an additional minute, then remove from heat.
7. Serve the beef stir-fry hot.

NUTRITIONAL INFORMATION:

Calories: 320 | **Protein:** 26 g | **Carbohydrates:** 10 g | **Dietary Fiber:** 2 g | **Sugars:** 4 g | **Fat:** 20 g | **Sodium:** 200 mg | **Potassium:** 400 mg | **Phosphorus:** 250 mg

Chicken Caesar Salad

(No Anchovies)

Yield: 1 serving | **Prep time:** 10 minutes | **Cook time:** 10 minutes

INGREDIENTS:

- 1 boneless, skinless chicken breast (about 6 oz)
- 2 cups chopped romaine lettuce
- 1 tablespoon olive oil
- 1/4 cup low-sodium Caesar dressing
- 2 tablespoons grated Parmesan cheese
- A pinch of black pepper
- Whole wheat croutons for garnish (optional)

DIRECTIONS:

1. Season the chicken breast with black pepper.
2. Heat olive oil in a skillet over medium heat. Add the chicken breast for 5 minutes on each side until fully cooked, and the internal temperature reaches 165°F (75°C). Let it cool slightly, and then slice it.
3. Toss the chopped romaine lettuce with the low-sodium Caesar dressing in a large bowl.
4. Add the sliced chicken breast to the salad.
5. Sprinkle with grated Parmesan cheese.
6. Garnish with whole wheat croutons if desired.
7. Serve the Chicken Caesar Salad immediately.

NUTRITIONAL INFORMATION:

Calories: 350 | **Protein:** 35 g | **Carbohydrates:** 8 g | **Dietary Fiber:** 2 g | **Sugars:** 3 g | **Fat:** 20 g | **Sodium:** 300 mg | **Potassium:** 500 mg | **Phosphorus:** 250 mg

Vegetable Sushi Rolls with Low-Sodium Soy Sauce

Yield: 1 serving | **Prep time:** 20 minutes | **Cook time:** 0 minutes

INGREDIENTS:

- 1 nori seaweed sheet
- 1/2 cup cooked sushi rice (cool to room temperature)
- 1/4 cucumber, julienned
- 1/4 avocado, sliced
- 1/4 carrot, julienned
- 1 tablespoon rice vinegar (optional for sushi rice)
- Low-sodium soy sauce for dipping
- Wasabi and pickled ginger for serving (optional)

DIRECTIONS:

1. Mix the rice vinegar into the cooked sushi rice for flavor.
2. Place the nori sheet on a bamboo sushi mat or parchment paper.
3. Spread the sushi rice evenly over the nori, leaving about 1/2 inch of space at the top.
4. Arrange the julienned cucumber, avocado slices, and carrot on the rice towards the bottom of the nori.
5. Carefully roll the sushi using the mat or parchment paper, tucking in the fillings as you move. Ensure the roll is tight and even.
6. Use a sharp, wet knife to slice the roll into 6-8 pieces.
7. Serve the vegetable sushi rolls with low-sodium soy sauce, wasabi, and pickled ginger optionally.

NUTRITIONAL INFORMATION:

Calories: 300 | **Protein:** 6 g | **Carbohydrates:** 45 g | **Dietary Fiber:** 5 g | **Sugars:** 3 g | **Fat:** 10 g | **Sodium:** 200 mg | **Potassium:** 400 mg | **Phosphorus:** 100 mg

Baked Salmon with Dill

Yield: 1 serving | **Prep time:** 5 minutes | **Cook time:** 15 minutes

INGREDIENTS:

- 1 salmon fillet (about 6 oz)
- 1 teaspoon olive oil
- A pinch of black pepper
- A pinch of dried dill or fresh dill, chopped
- Lemon slices for serving

DIRECTIONS:

1. Preheat your oven to 375°F (190°C).
2. Place the salmon fillet on a baking sheet lined with parchment paper.
3. Brush the salmon with olive oil and season with black pepper and dill.
4. Bake in the oven for about 15 minutes or until the salmon flakes easily with a fork.
5. Remove from the oven and let it rest for a few minutes.
6. Serve the baked salmon with lemon slices on the side.

NUTRITIONAL INFORMATION:

Calories: 280 | **Protein:** 35 g | **Carbohydrates:** 0 g | **Dietary Fiber:** 0 g | **Sugars:** 0 g | **Fat:** 15 g | **Sodium:** 70 mg | **Potassium:** 500 mg | **Phosphorus:** 300 mg

Stuffed Bell Peppers

(Low Potassium)

Yield: 1 serving | **Prep time:** 15 minutes | **Cook time:** 30 minutes

INGREDIENTS:

- 1 medium bell pepper
- 1/4 cup cooked white rice
- 2 oz lean ground turkey
- 1 tablespoon diced onion
- 1/4 cup low-sodium canned diced tomatoes
- 1 teaspoon olive oil
- A pinch of black pepper
- A pinch of garlic powder
- 1 tablespoon low-sodium cheese, shredded (optional)

DIRECTIONS:

1. Preheat your oven to 350°F (175°C).
2. Cut the top off the bell pepper and remove the seeds and membranes.
3. In a skillet, heat olive oil over medium heat. Add the diced onion and ground turkey. Cook until the turkey is browned.
4. Stir in the cooked rice, low-sodium diced tomatoes, black pepper, and garlic powder. Cook for an additional 2-3 minutes.
5. Stuff the mixture into the bell pepper.
6. Place the stuffed pepper in a baking dish and cover with foil.
7. Bake in the oven for 25-30 minutes or until the pepper is tender.
8. Sprinkle shredded low-sodium cheese on top of the pepper during the last 5 minutes of baking if using.
9. Serve the stuffed bell pepper hot.

NUTRITIONAL INFORMATION:

Calories: 250 | **Protein:** 15 g | **Carbohydrates:** 20 g | **Dietary Fiber:** 3 g | **Sugars:** 5 g | **Fat:** 12 g | **Sodium:** 100 mg | **Potassium:** 300 mg | **Phosphorus:** 150 mg

Egg White Scramble with Asparagus

Yield: 1 serving | **Prep time:** 5 minutes | **Cook time:** 10 minutes

INGREDIENTS:

- 3 egg whites
- 1/2 cup chopped asparagus
- 1 tablespoon diced onion
- 1 teaspoon olive oil
- A pinch of black pepper
- A pinch of garlic powder
- Fresh herbs (like parsley or chives) for garnish (optional)

DIRECTIONS:

1. Heat olive oil in a non-stick skillet over medium heat.
2. Add the diced onion and chopped asparagus to the skillet. Sauté for about 3-4 minutes until the asparagus is tender-crisp.
3. Whisk the egg whites, black pepper, and garlic powder in a bowl.
4. Pour the egg whites into the skillet with the asparagus and onion.
5. Cook while gently stirring until the egg whites are set and fully cooked, about 3-5 minutes.
6. Remove from heat and transfer to a plate.
7. Garnish with fresh herbs if desired.
8. Serve the egg white scramble hot.

NUTRITIONAL INFORMATION:

Calories: 120 | **Protein:** 15 g | **Carbohydrates:** 4 g | **Dietary Fiber:** 1 g | **Sugars:** 2 g | **Fat:** 5 g | **Sodium:** 170 mg | **Potassium:** 300 mg | **Phosphorus:** 100 mg

Tofu and Broccoli Stir-Fry

Yield: 1 serving | **Prep time:** 10 minutes | **Cook time:** 10 minutes

INGREDIENTS:

- 1/2 cup firm tofu, cubed
- 1 cup broccoli florets
- 1 tablespoon olive oil
- 1 clove garlic, minced
- 1 teaspoon ginger, grated
- 1 tablespoon low-sodium soy sauce
- A pinch of black pepper
- 1 teaspoon sesame seeds (optional)
- 1/4 cup water or low-sodium vegetable broth

DIRECTIONS:

1. Press the tofu with a paper towel to remove excess moisture. Cut into small cubes.
2. Heat olive oil in a skillet or wok over medium-high heat. Add the minced garlic, grated ginger, and sauté for about 1 minute.
3. Add the tofu cubes to the skillet. Cook, stirring occasionally, until the tofu is golden brown on all sides, about 3-4 minutes.
4. Add the broccoli florets and water or vegetable broth. Cover and let steam for 2-3 minutes or until the broccoli is bright green and tender.
5. Uncover and stir in the low-sodium soy sauce and black pepper. Cook for an additional 1-2 minutes.
6. Sprinkle with sesame seeds if using.
7. Serve the tofu and broccoli stir-fry hot.

NUTRITIONAL INFORMATION:

Calories: 280 | **Protein:** 18 g | **Carbohydrates:** 15 g | **Dietary Fiber:** 4 g | **Sugars:** 3 g | **Fat:** 18 g | **Sodium:** 300 mg | **Potassium:** 450 mg | **Phosphorus:** 200 mg

Vegetarian Chili with Kidney Beans

Yield: 1 serving | **Prep time:** 10 minutes | **Cook time:** 30 minutes

INGREDIENTS:

- 1/2 cup canned low-sodium kidney beans drained and rinsed
- 1/2 cup canned low-sodium diced tomatoes
- 1/4 cup diced bell pepper
- 1/4 cup diced onion
- 1 clove garlic, minced
- 1 teaspoon olive oil
- 1/2 teaspoon chili powder (adjust to taste)
- A pinch of cumin
- A pinch of black pepper
- 1/2 cup water or low-sodium vegetable broth
- Fresh cilantro for garnish (optional)

DIRECTIONS:

1. Heat olive oil in a pot over medium heat. Add the diced onion and garlic, and sauté until the onion is translucent.

2. Add the diced bell pepper to the pot and cook for 3 minutes.

3. Stir in the chili powder, cumin, and black pepper.

4. Add the low-sodium kidney beans and diced tomatoes to the pot. Pour in the water or vegetable broth.

5. Bring the chili to a boil, then reduce the heat to low and simmer, covered, for about 25 minutes, stirring occasionally.

6. Once the chili has thickened to your liking, remove it from heat.

7. Serve the chili hot, garnished with fresh cilantro if desired.

NUTRITIONAL INFORMATION:

Calories: 200 | **Protein:** 10 g | **Carbohydrates:** 30 g | **Dietary Fiber:** 8 g | **Sugars:** 5 g | **Fat:** 5 g | **Sodium:** 150 mg | **Potassium:** 400 mg | **Phosphorus:** 150 mg

CHAPTER 7

Dinner Recipes

—

Asian-Style Tofu Stir-Fry with Vegetables

Yield: 1 serving | **Prep time:** 15 minutes | **Cook time:** 10 minutes

INGREDIENTS:

- 4 oz firm tofu, pressed and cubed
- 1/2 cup sliced bell peppers (mixed colors)
- 1/4 cup sliced carrots
- 1/4 cup broccoli florets
- 1 tablespoon olive oil
- 1 clove garlic, minced
- 1 teaspoon grated ginger
- 1 tablespoon low-sodium soy sauce
- 1 teaspoon sesame oil
- 1/2 teaspoon rice vinegar
- A pinch of black pepper
- Fresh cilantro for garnish
- Sesame seeds for garnish

DIRECTIONS:

1. Heat olive oil in a large skillet or wok over medium-high heat.

2. Add garlic and ginger to the skillet and sauté for about 1 minute until fragrant.

3. Increase heat to high and add the tofu cubes. Stir-fry for 2-3 minutes until lightly browned.

4. Add the sliced bell peppers, carrots, and broccoli to the skillet. Continue to stir-fry for another 5 minutes until the vegetables are tender-crisp.

5. Whisk together low-sodium soy sauce, sesame oil, and rice vinegar in a small bowl. Pour this mixture over the tofu and vegetables in the skillet. Stir well to combine and heat through for another minute.

6. Season with black pepper to taste.

7. Serve the stir-fry garnished with fresh cilantro and sesame seeds.

NUTRITIONAL INFORMATION:

Calories: 320 | **Protein:** 12 g | **Carbohydrates:** 15 g | **Dietary Fiber:** 4 g | **Sugars:** 6 g | **Fat:** 24 g | **Sodium:** 320 mg | **Potassium:** 400 mg | **Phosphorus:** 150 mg

Baked Cod with Parsley Pesto

Yield: 1 serving | **Prep time:** 10 minutes | **Cook time:** 15 minutes

INGREDIENTS:

- 1 cod fillet (about 6 oz)
- 1/4 cup fresh parsley leaves
- 1 tablespoon olive oil
- 1 clove garlic
- 2 tablespoons grated Parmesan cheese (optional; use low-phosphorus if needed)
- A pinch of black pepper
- Lemon slices for garnish

DIRECTIONS:

1. Preheat your oven to 400°F (200°C).
2. In a food processor, combine the parsley leaves, olive oil, garlic, Parmesan cheese (if using), and black pepper. Pulse until you achieve a pesto-like consistency.
3. Place the cod fillet on a baking sheet lined with parchment paper.
4. Spread the parsley pesto evenly over the top of the cod fillet.
5. Bake in the oven for about 15 minutes or until the fish flakes easily with a fork.
6. Remove the cod from the oven and let it rest for a few minutes.
7. Serve the baked cod garnished with lemon slices.

NUTRITIONAL INFORMATION:

Calories: 250 | **Protein:** 28 g | **Carbohydrates:** 1 g | **Dietary Fiber:** 0 g | **Sugars:** 0 g | **Fat:** 14 g | **Sodium:** 120 mg | **Potassium:** 500 mg | **Phosphorus:** 250 mg

Low-Sodium Beef Stroganoff

Yield: 1 serving | **Prep time:** 15 minutes | **Cook time:** 20 minutes

INGREDIENTS:

- 4 oz lean beef sirloin, thinly sliced
- 1/2 cup sliced mushrooms
- 1/4 cup diced onion
- 1 clove garlic, minced
- 1/2 cup low-sodium beef broth
- 1 tablespoon olive oil
- 2 tablespoons sour cream (use low-sodium, if available)
- 1/2 teaspoon Dijon mustard
- A pinch of black pepper
- 1/2 cup cooked egg noodles (use low-sodium, if available)

DIRECTIONS:

1. Heat olive oil in a skillet over medium-high heat. Add the beef slices and cook until browned on both sides. Remove the beef from the skillet and set aside.
2. Add the onions and garlic, and sauté until translucent in the same skillet.
3. Add the mushrooms to the skillet and cook until they begin to release their moisture.
4. Return the beef to the skillet and add the low-sodium beef broth. Bring to a simmer and cook for about 5 minutes.
5. Stir in the sour cream and Dijon mustard. Heat through, but do not boil, to avoid curdling the sour cream.
6. Season with black pepper to taste.
7. Serve the beef stroganoff over the cooked egg noodles.

NUTRITIONAL INFORMATION:

Calories: 400 | **Protein:** 30 g | **Carbohydrates:** 20 g | **Dietary Fiber:** 2 g | **Sugars:** 3 g | **Fat:** 22 g | **Sodium:** 150 mg | **Potassium:** 650 mg | **Phosphorus:** 250 mg

Lemon Pepper Baked Salmon

Yield: 1 serving | **Prep time:** 5 minutes | **Cook time:** 15 minutes

INGREDIENTS:

- 1 salmon fillet (about 6 oz)
- Juice of 1/2 lemon
- 1 teaspoon olive oil
- 1/2 teaspoon lemon pepper seasoning
- A pinch of dried dill (optional)
- Lemon slices for garnish

DIRECTIONS:

1. Preheat your oven to 375°F (190°C).
2. Place the salmon fillet on a baking sheet lined with parchment paper.
3. Drizzle olive oil and lemon juice over the salmon.
4. Sprinkle the lemon pepper seasoning and dried dill over the salmon.
5. Bake in the oven for about 15 minutes or until the salmon flakes easily with a fork.
6. Remove from the oven and let it rest for a few minutes.
7. Garnish with lemon slices before serving.

NUTRITIONAL INFORMATION:

Calories: 300 | **Protein:** 34 g | **Carbohydrates:** 1 g | **Dietary Fiber:** 0 g | **Sugars:** 0 g | **Fat:** 18 g | **Sodium:** 120 mg | **Potassium:** 830 mg | **Phosphorus:** 400 mg

Eggplant Parmesan with Low-Phosphorus Cheese

Yield: 1 serving | **Prep time:** 15 minutes | **Cook time:** 30 minutes

INGREDIENTS:

- 1 medium eggplant, sliced into 1/2-inch rounds
- 1/2 cup low-sodium marinara sauce
- 1/4 cup shredded low-phosphorus mozzarella cheese (consult with a dietitian for appropriate brands)
- 1 tablespoon grated Parmesan cheese (low-phosphorus, if available)
- 1 teaspoon olive oil
- A pinch of dried oregano
- A pinch of black pepper
- Fresh basil for garnish

DIRECTIONS:

1. Preheat your oven to 375°F (190°C).
2. Brush both sides of the eggplant slices with olive oil and place them on a baking sheet.
3. Bake the eggplant slices for about 20 minutes, turning halfway through, until they are tender and slightly golden.
4. Spread a small amount of marinara sauce on the bottom of a baking dish.
5. Layer the baked eggplant slices in the dish, topping each slice with marinara sauce.
6. Sprinkle the shredded low-phosphorus mozzarella and grated Parmesan cheese over the eggplant slices.
7. Season with dried oregano and black pepper.
8. Bake in the oven for 10 minutes or until the cheese is melted and bubbly.
9. Garnish with fresh basil leaves before serving.

NUTRITIONAL INFORMATION:

Calories: 250 | **Protein:** 12 g | **Carbohydrates:** 20 g | **Dietary Fiber:** 8 g | **Sugars:** 12 g | **Fat:** 14 g | **Sodium:** 300 mg | **Potassium:** 400 mg | **Phosphorus:** 150 mg

Quinoa Stuffed Bell Peppers

Yield: 1 serving | **Prep time:** 15 minutes | **Cook time:** 30 minutes

INGREDIENTS:

- 1 large bell pepper, halved and deseeded
- 1/4 cup cooked quinoa
- 1/4 cup canned low-sodium black beans, rinsed and drained
- 1/4 cup diced tomatoes
- 1 tablespoon diced onion
- 1 clove garlic, minced
- 1/4 teaspoon cumin
- 1/4 teaspoon chili powder
- 1 teaspoon olive oil
- 2 tablespoons shredded low-sodium cheese (optional)
- Fresh cilantro for garnish

DIRECTIONS:

1. Preheat your oven to 350°F (175°C).
2. In a skillet, heat olive oil over medium heat. Add onion and garlic, and sauté until softened.
3. Stir in the cooked quinoa, black beans, diced tomatoes, cumin, and chili powder. Cook for about 5 minutes, until the mixture is heated through.
4. Spoon the quinoa mixture into the bell pepper halves.
5. Place the stuffed peppers in a baking dish and cover with foil.
6. Bake in the oven for 25-30 minutes or until the peppers are tender.
7. If using cheese, sprinkle it over the peppers in the last 5 minutes of baking.
8. Garnish with fresh cilantro before serving.

NUTRITIONAL INFORMATION:

Calories: 280 | **Protein:** 10 g | **Carbohydrates:** 40 g | **Dietary Fiber:** 8 g | **Sugars:** 5 g | **Fat:** 10 g | **Sodium:** 200 mg | **Potassium:** 500 mg | **Phosphorus:** 150 mg

Kidney-Friendly Turkey Meatloaf

Yield: 1 serving | **Prep time:** 15 minutes | **Cook time:** 45 minutes

INGREDIENTS:

- 4 oz ground turkey
- 1/4 cup breadcrumbs (low sodium)
- 2 tablespoons milk (use non-dairy for lower phosphorus)
- 1 tablespoon grated onion
- 1 clove garlic, minced
- 1 egg white
- 1 teaspoon olive oil
- A pinch of black pepper
- 1 tablespoon low-sodium ketchup for topping

DIRECTIONS:

1. Preheat your oven to 375°F (190°C).
2. Combine the ground turkey, breadcrumbs, milk, grated onion, minced garlic, egg white, and black pepper in a bowl. Mix until well combined.
3. Grease a small baking dish or loaf pan with olive oil.
4. Shape the turkey mixture into a loaf and place it in the prepared baking dish.
5. Spread the low-sodium ketchup over the top of the meatloaf.
6. Bake in the preheated oven for about 45 minutes or until the meatloaf is cooked and reaches an internal temperature of 165°F (74°C).
7. Let the meatloaf rest briefly before slicing and serving.

NUTRITIONAL INFORMATION:

Calories: 320 | **Protein:** 28 g | **Carbohydrates:** 15 g | **Dietary Fiber:** 1 g | **Sugars:** 4 g | **Fat:** 16 g | **Sodium:** 200 mg | **Potassium:** 350 mg | **Phosphorus:** 180 mg

Oven-Baked Tilapia With Fresh Herbs

Yield: 1 serving | **Prep time:** 10 minutes | **Cook time:** 15 minutes

INGREDIENTS:

- 1 tilapia fillet (about 6 oz)
- 1 teaspoon olive oil
- 1 tablespoon chopped fresh parsley
- 1 teaspoon chopped fresh dill
- 1 clove garlic, minced
- A pinch of black pepper
- Lemon slices for garnish

DIRECTIONS:

1. Preheat your oven to 400°F (200°C).
2. Place the tilapia fillet on an aluminum foil large enough to fold over and seal.
3. Brush the tilapia with olive oil and sprinkle the chopped parsley, dill, minced garlic, and black pepper evenly over the top.
4. Place a few lemon slices on top of the herbs.
5. Fold the foil around the tilapia to seal it, creating a pouch.
6. Bake in the oven for about 15 minutes or until the fish flakes easily with a fork.
7. Carefully open the foil pouch (watch for steam), and transfer the tilapia to a serving plate.
8. Garnish with additional fresh herbs and lemon slices before serving.

NUTRITIONAL INFORMATION:

Calories: 200 | **Protein:** 23 g | **Carbohydrates:** 2 g | **Dietary Fiber:** 0.5 g | **Sugars:** 0 g | **Fat:** 11 g | **Sodium:** 60 mg | **Potassium:** 500 mg | **Phosphorus:** 250 mg

Oven-Baked Sweet Potato with Cinnamon
(Small Portion)

Yield: 1 serving | **Prep time:** 5 minutes | **Cook time:** 25 minutes

INGREDIENTS:

- 1 small sweet potato (about 4 oz)
- 1/2 teaspoon olive oil
- A pinch of cinnamon
- A pinch of nutmeg (optional)
- A sprinkle of brown sugar substitute (optional for those monitoring blood sugar levels)

DIRECTIONS:

1. Preheat your oven to 400°F (200°C).
2. Wash the sweet potato thoroughly and pat dry. Prick the sweet potato several times with a fork to allow steam to escape during baking.
3. Rub the outside of the sweet potato with olive oil, then sprinkle with cinnamon and nutmeg, if using.
4. Place the sweet potato on a baking sheet lined with parchment paper.
5. Bake in the preheated oven for about 25 minutes or until the sweet potato is tender when pierced with a fork.
6. Remove from the oven and let cool for a few minutes. If desired, split the top open and sprinkle a slight brown sugar substitute for added sweetness.
7. Serve warm and enjoy the comforting flavors.

NUTRITIONAL INFORMATION:

Calories: 90 | **Protein:** 2 g | **Carbohydrates:** 20 g | **Dietary Fiber:** 3 g | **Sugars:** 5 g | **Fat:** 1 g | **Sodium:** 30 mg | **Potassium:** 400 mg | **Phosphorus:** 60 mg

Lentil Soup with Carrots and Celery

Yield: 1 serving | **Prep time:** 10 minutes | **Cook time:** 30 minutes

INGREDIENTS:

- 1/2 cup dried lentils, rinsed
- 2 cups low-sodium vegetable broth
- 1/4 cup diced carrots
- 1/4 cup diced celery
- 1 tablespoon diced onion
- 1 clove garlic, minced
- 1/2 teaspoon olive oil
- A pinch of dried thyme
- A pinch of black pepper
- 1 bay leaf (optional)

DIRECTIONS:

1. Heat olive oil in a medium-sized pot over medium heat. Add diced onion and garlic, and sauté until softened, about 2-3 minutes.
2. Add diced carrots and celery to the pot, sautéing for 3-4 minutes until slightly softening.
3. Stir in the rinsed lentils, low-sodium vegetable broth, thyme, black pepper, and bay leaf if using. Bring to a boil.
4. Once boiling, reduce heat to low, cover, and simmer for about 25-30 minutes or until the lentils are tender.
5. Remove the bay leaf and adjust the seasoning to taste.
6. Serve the soup hot, garnished with a sprinkle of fresh herbs if desired.

NUTRITIONAL INFORMATION:

Calories: 240 | **Protein:** 15 g | **Carbohydrates:** 40 g | **Dietary Fiber:** 15 g | **Sugars:** 4 g | **Fat:** 2 g | **Sodium:** 100 mg | **Potassium:** 600 mg | **Phosphorus:** 200 mg

Cauliflower Fried Rice

Yield: 1 serving | **Prep time:** 10 minutes | **Cook time:** 10 minutes

INGREDIENTS:

- 2 cups cauliflower rice (grated cauliflower)
- 1/4 cup diced carrots
- 1/4 cup peas (use fresh or frozen, thawed)
- 2 tablespoons chopped green onions
- 1 clove garlic, minced
- 1 egg, beaten (or use two egg whites for lower phosphorus)
- 1 tablespoon olive oil
- 1 tablespoon low-sodium soy sauce
- A pinch of black pepper
- Fresh cilantro for garnish

DIRECTIONS:

1. Heat olive oil in a large skillet or wok over medium heat. Add the minced garlic and sauté until fragrant, about 1 minute.
2. Add the diced carrots and peas to the skillet. Stir-fry for about 2-3 minutes until the vegetables are tender.
3. Increase the heat to medium-high and add the cauliflower rice. Stir-fry for about 5 minutes until the cauliflower is tender and slightly crispy.
4. Push the cauliflower mixture to the side of the skillet and add the beaten egg to the empty side. Scramble the egg, mixing it with the vegetables once cooked.
5. Drizzle the low-sodium soy sauce over the cauliflower mixture and season with black pepper. Stir well to combine.
6. Cook for an additional 2 minutes, then remove from heat.
7. Serve the cauliflower fried rice garnished with chopped green onions and fresh cilantro.

NUTRITIONAL INFORMATION:

Calories: 280 | **Protein:** 12 g | **Carbohydrates:** 18 g | **Dietary Fiber:** 5 g | **Sugars:** 6 g | **Fat:** 18 g | **Sodium:** 320 mg | **Potassium:** 600 mg | **Phosphorus:** 150 mg

Pan-Seared Pork Chops with Apples

Yield: 1 serving | **Prep time:** 10 minutes | **Cook time:** 20 minutes

INGREDIENTS:

- 1 (6 oz) boneless pork chop, trimmed of fat
- 1/2 apple, sliced
- 1/2 teaspoon olive oil
- A pinch of black pepper
- A pinch of dried thyme
- 1/4 cup low-sodium chicken broth
- 1 teaspoon balsamic vinegar

DIRECTIONS:

1. Heat olive oil in a skillet over medium-high heat.
2. Season the pork chop with black pepper and thyme. Place in the skillet and cook for about 4-5 minutes on each side or until browned and cooked to an internal temperature of 145°F (63°C).
3. Remove the pork chop from the skillet and set aside, covering with foil to keep warm.
4. Add sliced apples, low-sodium chicken broth, and balsamic vinegar in the same skillet. Cook over medium heat, stirring occasionally, until the apples are tender and the sauce has thickened slightly about 5-7 minutes.
5. Serve the pork chop topped with the cooked apples and drizzled with the pan sauce.

NUTRITIONAL INFORMATION:

Calories: 280 | **Protein:** 25 g | **Carbohydrates:** 15 g | **Dietary Fiber:** 2 g | **Sugars:** 10 g | **Fat:** 12 g | **Sodium:** 70 mg | **Potassium:** 550 mg | **Phosphorus:** 220 mg

Garlic Shrimp with Zucchini Noodles

Yield: 1 serving | **Prep time:** 15 minutes | **Cook time:** 10 minutes

INGREDIENTS:

- 6 large shrimp, peeled and deveined
- 1 large zucchini, spiralized into noodles
- 1 tablespoon olive oil
- 2 cloves garlic, minced
- A pinch of red pepper flakes (optional)
- A pinch of black pepper
- Fresh parsley, chopped for garnish
- Lemon wedges for serving

DIRECTIONS:

1. Heat olive oil in a large skillet over medium heat.
2. Add minced garlic and red pepper flakes to the skillet and sauté for about 1 minute until fragrant.
3. Increase the heat to medium-high and add the shrimp to the skillet. Season with black pepper.
4. Cook the shrimp on each side for 2-3 minutes until they turn pink and opaque.
5. Remove the shrimp from the skillet and set aside.
6. Add the zucchini noodles and sauté in the same skillet for 2-3 minutes or until tender.
7. Return the shrimp to the skillet and toss with the zucchini noodles to heat through.
8. Serve the garlic shrimp with zucchini noodles garnished with chopped parsley and lemon wedges on the side.

NUTRITIONAL INFORMATION:

Calories: 250 | **Protein:** 18 g | **Carbohydrates:** 10 g | **Dietary Fiber:** 2 g | **Sugars:** 4 g | **Fat:** 16 g | **Sodium:** 120 mg | **Potassium:** 600 mg | **Phosphorus:** 200 mg

Low-Sodium Chicken Noodle Soup

Yield: 1 serving | **Prep time:** 10 minutes | **Cook time:** 20 minutes

INGREDIENTS:

- 4 oz chicken breast, cooked and shredded
- 1 cup low-sodium chicken broth
- 1/2 cup water
- 1/4 cup sliced carrots
- 1/4 cup diced celery
- 1/4 cup cooked egg noodles
- 1 tablespoon chopped onion
- 1 clove garlic, minced
- A pinch of dried thyme
- A pinch of black pepper
- Fresh parsley for garnish

DIRECTIONS:

1. In a large pot, combine low-sodium chicken broth and water. Bring to a simmer over medium heat.
2. Add sliced carrots, diced celery, chopped onion, and minced garlic to the pot. Simmer for about 10 minutes or until the vegetables are tender.
3. Add the cooked, shredded chicken breast and egg noodles to the pot. Stir well.
4. Season the soup with dried thyme and black pepper. Adjust seasoning according to taste, keeping sodium intake in mind.
5. Simmer the soup for 5-10 minutes, allowing all the flavors to meld together.
6. Remove from heat Once the soup and the vegetables are tender.
7. Serve the chicken noodle soup hot, garnished with fresh parsley.

NUTRITIONAL INFORMATION:

Calories: 220 | **Protein:** 25 g | **Carbohydrates:** 15 g | **Dietary Fiber:** 2 g | **Sugars:** 3 g | **Fat:** 5 g | **Sodium:** 100 mg | **Potassium:** 400 mg | **Phosphorus:** 220 mg

One-Pan Balsamic Chicken and Veggies

Yield: 1 serving | **Prep time:** 10 minutes | **Cook time:** 20 minutes

INGREDIENTS:

- 1 (6 oz) chicken breast, pounded to even thickness
- 1/2 cup cherry tomatoes, halved
- 1/2 cup broccoli florets
- 1/2 cup sliced carrots
- 2 tablespoons balsamic vinegar
- 1 tablespoon olive oil
- 1 clove garlic, minced
- A pinch of dried basil
- A pinch of dried oregano
- A pinch of black pepper

DIRECTIONS:

1. Preheat your oven to 400°F (200°C).
2. Mix balsamic vinegar, olive oil, minced garlic, basil, oregano, and black pepper in a bowl.
3. Place the chicken breast in the center of a baking sheet.
4. Arrange the cherry tomatoes, broccoli florets, and sliced carrots around the chicken on the baking sheet.
5. Pour the balsamic mixture over the chicken and vegetables, ensuring everything is well coated.
6. Bake in the preheated oven for 20 minutes or until the chicken is cooked through (reaching an internal temperature of 165°F) and the vegetables are tender.
7. Remove from the oven and let it rest for a few minutes before serving.

NUTRITIONAL INFORMATION:

Calories: 350 | **Protein:** 26 g | **Carbohydrates:** 18 g | **Dietary Fiber:** 4 g | **Sugars:** 10 g | **Fat:** 18 g | **Sodium:** 150 mg | **Potassium:** 700 mg | **Phosphorus:** 250 mg

Sautéed Tilapia with Lemon and Herbs

Yield: 1 serving | **Prep time:** 5 minutes | **Cook time:** 10 minutes

INGREDIENTS:

- 1 tilapia fillet (about 6 oz)
- 1 teaspoon olive oil
- Juice of 1/2 lemon
- 1/2 teaspoon dried parsley
- 1/2 teaspoon dried dill
- A pinch of black pepper
- Lemon slices for garnish

DIRECTIONS:

1. Heat olive oil in a non-stick skillet over medium heat.
2. Season the tilapia fillet with black pepper, parsley, and dill on both sides.
3. Once the skillet is hot, place the tilapia fillet in the skillet.
4. Cook on one side for 4-5 minutes, then flip the fillet carefully.
5. Squeeze the lemon juice over the fillet after flipping.
6. Continue cooking for another 4-5 minutes or until the fish is opaque and flakes easily with a fork.
7. Transfer the cooked tilapia to a serving plate and garnish with lemon slices.
8. Serve hot, enjoying the fresh, citrusy flavors.

NUTRITIONAL INFORMATION:

Calories: 200 | **Protein:** 23 g | **Carbohydrates:** 2 g | **Dietary Fiber:** 0 g | **Sugars:** 0 g | **Fat:** 10 g | **Sodium:** 60 mg | **Potassium:** 350 mg | **Phosphorus:** 200 mg

Sautéed Lemon Garlic Scallops

Yield: 1 serving | **Prep time:** 5 minutes | **Cook time:** 10 minutes

INGREDIENTS:

- 4 large sea scallops
- 1 teaspoon olive oil
- 1 clove garlic, minced
- Juice of 1/2 lemon
- A pinch of black pepper
- Fresh parsley, chopped for garnish

DIRECTIONS:

1. Pat the scallops dry with paper towels to ensure proper searing.
2. Heat olive oil in a non-stick skillet over medium-high heat.
3. Once the oil is hot, add the scallops to the skillet, taking care not to overcrowd them. Cook without moving them for about 2 minutes or until a golden crust forms on the bottom.
4. Flip the scallops and add the minced garlic to the skillet. Cook for 2 minutes or until the other side is golden and the scallops are nearly opaque in the center.
5. Squeeze the lemon juice over the scallops and sprinkle with black pepper. Stir gently to mix the lemon juice and garlic around the scallops.
6. Remove from heat and transfer the scallops to a serving plate. Pour any remaining garlic lemon sauce from the skillet over the scallops.
7. Garnish with fresh parsley before serving.

NUTRITIONAL INFORMATION:

Calories: 150 | **Protein:** 14 g | **Carbohydrates:** 4 g | **Dietary Fiber:** 0 g | **Sugars:** 0 g | **Fat:** 8 g | **Sodium:** 200 mg | **Potassium:** 350 mg | **Phosphorus:** 200 mg

Low-Sodium Tomato Basil Pasta

Yield: 1 serving | **Prep time:** 10 minutes | **Cook time:** 15 minutes

INGREDIENTS:

- 1 cup cooked whole wheat pasta
- 1/2 cup cherry tomatoes, halved
- 1 tablespoon olive oil
- 1 clove garlic, minced
- 1/4 cup fresh basil leaves, chopped
- Salt substitute and black pepper, to taste
- 1 tablespoon grated Parmesan cheese (optional)

DIRECTIONS:

1. Cook the pasta according to package instructions without adding salt. Drain and set aside.
2. In a skillet over medium heat, heat the olive oil and sauté the garlic until fragrant, about 1 minute.
3. Add the cherry tomatoes to the skillet and cook until they are soft and the skins begin to wrinkle about 5 minutes.
4. Toss in the cooked pasta and chopped basil—season with a salt substitute and black pepper to taste. Stir well to combine all the ingredients.
5. Cook for an additional 2-3 minutes, just until the pasta is heated through.
6. Serve hot, garnished with grated Parmesan cheese if desired.

NUTRITIONAL INFORMATION:

Calories: 320 | **Protein:** 10 g | **Carbohydrates:** 45 g | **Dietary Fiber:** 7 g | **Sugars:** 4 g | **Fat:** 12 g | **Sodium:** 70 mg | **Potassium:** 300 mg | **Phosphorus:** 200 mg

Barley and Vegetable Stew

Yield: 1 serving | **Prep time:** 10 minutes | **Cook time:** 45 minutes

INGREDIENTS:

- 1/4 cup pearl barley, rinsed
- 1 cup low-sodium vegetable broth
- 1/4 cup diced carrots
- 1/4 cup diced celery
- 1/4 cup chopped onions
- 1/2 cup chopped tomatoes
- 1 clove garlic, minced
- 1/2 teaspoon olive oil
- A pinch of dried thyme
- A pinch of black pepper
- 1 bay leaf (optional)
- 1/2 cup water (adjust as needed)

DIRECTIONS:

1. Heat olive oil in a pot over medium heat. Add onions and garlic, sautéing until softened, about 2-3 minutes.
2. Add carrots and celery to the pot and continue to sauté for another 5 minutes.
3. Stir in the pearl barley, chopped tomatoes, low-sodium vegetable broth, thyme, black pepper, and bay leaf if using.
4. Bring the mixture to a boil, then reduce heat to low, cover, and simmer for about 40 minutes, or until the barley is tender and the stew has thickened. Add water as necessary to adjust the consistency according to your preference.
5. Remove the bay leaf and adjust the seasoning to taste. Once the barley is cooked and the vegetables are tender.
6. Serve the barley and vegetable stew hot, garnished with fresh herbs if desired.

NUTRITIONAL INFORMATION:

Calories: 250 | **Protein:** 6 g | **Carbohydrates:** 55 g | **Dietary Fiber:** 11 g | **Sugars:** 5 g | **Fat:** 3 g | **Sodium:** 200 mg | **Potassium:** 400 mg | **Phosphorus:** 150 mg

Roasted Turkey Breast with Rosemary

Yield: 1 serving | **Prep time:** 10 minutes | **Cook time:** 60 minutes

INGREDIENTS:

- 1 (6-ounce) turkey breast
- 1/2 tablespoon olive oil
- 1/2 teaspoon dried rosemary
- A pinch of black pepper
- 1/2 garlic clove, minced

DIRECTIONS:

1. Preheat your oven to 350°F (175°C).

2. Rub the turkey breast with olive oil, then season with the minced garlic, dried rosemary, and black pepper.

3. Place the seasoned turkey breast in a roasting pan.

4. Roast in the oven for approximately 60 minutes or until the turkey is fully cooked and the juices clear. The internal temperature should reach 165°F (74°C) when checked with a meat thermometer.

5. Once cooked, remove the turkey breast from the oven and let it rest for a few minutes before slicing to serve.

NUTRITIONAL INFORMATION:

Calories: 340 | **Protein:** 50g | **Carbohydrates:** 1g | **Dietary Fiber:** 0g | **Sugars:** 0g | **Fat:** 14g | **Sodium:** 125mg | **Potassium:** 500mg | **Phosphorus:** 400mg

Fish Tacos with Cabbage Slaw

Yield: 1 serving | **Prep time:** 20 minutes | **Cook time:** 10 minutes

INGREDIENTS:

- 1 (4 oz) white fish fillet (such as tilapia, cod, or halibut)
- 1 teaspoon olive oil
- Juice of 1/2 lime
- A pinch of chili powder
- A pinch of cumin
- A pinch of black pepper
- 2 small corn tortillas
- For the cabbage slaw:
- - 1/2 cup shredded cabbage
- - 1 tablespoon diced red onion
- - 1 tablespoon chopped cilantro
- - 1 teaspoon olive oil
- - 1 teaspoon apple cider vinegar
- - Juice of 1/4 lime
- - A pinch of black pepper

DIRECTIONS:

1. Preheat the grill or a grill pan over medium heat.

2. Mix lime juice, chili powder, cumin, and black pepper in a small bowl. Brush the fish fillet with olive oil and rub the lime juice mixture over both sides.

3. Grill the fish for 4-5 minutes on each side or until it flakes easily with a fork. Remove from heat and let it rest for a minute before flaking the fish into small pieces with a fork.

4. While the fish is cooking, prepare the cabbage slaw by mixing shredded cabbage, red onion, cilantro, olive oil, apple cider vinegar, lime juice, and black pepper in a bowl.

5. Warm the corn tortillas on the grill or pan for 30 seconds on each side.

6. Assemble the tacos by dividing the flaked fish evenly between the two tortillas. Top with the cabbage slaw.

7. Serve the fish tacos with a wedge of lime.

NUTRITIONAL INFORMATION:

Calories: 350 | **Protein:** 24 g | **Carbohydrates:** 35 g | **Dietary Fiber:** 5 g | **Sugars:** 3 g | **Fat:** 15 g | **Sodium:** 150 mg | **Potassium:** 500 mg | **Phosphorus:** 250 mg

Grilled Portobello Mushrooms

Yield: 1 serving | **Prep time:** 5 minutes | **Cook time:** 10 minutes

INGREDIENTS:

- 1 large Portobello mushroom cap
- 1 teaspoon olive oil
- A pinch of black pepper
- 1/2 teaspoon balsamic vinegar
- 1/2 garlic clove, minced

DIRECTIONS:

1. Preheat the grill to medium-high heat.
2. Clean the mushroom with a damp cloth and remove the stem.
3. Mix olive oil, balsamic vinegar, minced garlic, and black pepper in a small bowl. Brush both sides of the mushroom cap with the mixture.
4. Place the mushroom on the grill, gill side down, and cook for about 5 minutes. Flip the mushroom and grill for another 5 minutes or until it is tender and cooked.
5. Remove from grill and serve immediately.

NUTRITIONAL INFORMATION:

Calories: 60 | **Protein:** 2g | **Carbohydrates:** 4g | **Dietary Fiber:** 1g | **Sugars:** 2g | **Fat:** 4g | **Sodium:** 5mg | **Potassium:** 300mg | **Phosphorus:** 50mg

Pumpkin and Carrot Soup

Yield: 1 serving | **Prep time:** 10 minutes | **Cook time:** 30 minutes

INGREDIENTS:

- 1/2 cup pumpkin puree (fresh or canned without added sugar)
- 1/4 cup carrots, peeled and diced
- 1 cup low-sodium vegetable broth
- 1 tablespoon onion, finely chopped
- 1 clove garlic, minced
- 1/2 teaspoon olive oil
- A pinch of ground nutmeg
- A pinch of ground cinnamon
- Salt substitute and black pepper to taste
- Fresh parsley for garnish

DIRECTIONS:

1. Heat the olive oil in a saucepan over medium heat. Add the onions, garlic, and sauté until translucent and fragrant, about 2-3 minutes.
2. Add the diced carrots to the saucepan and cook for another 5 minutes, stirring occasionally.
3. Stir in the pumpkin puree and low-sodium vegetable broth. Bring the mixture to a simmer.
4. Season with ground nutmeg, cinnamon, salt substitute, and black pepper. Cover and simmer on low heat for about 20 minutes or until the carrots are tender.
5. Use an immersion blender to puree the soup directly in the pot until smooth. Alternatively, you can carefully transfer the soup to a blender to puree and then return it to the pot.
6. Heat the soup through, adjust seasoning if necessary, and remove from heat.
7. Serve hot, garnished with fresh parsley.

NUTRITIONAL INFORMATION:

Calories: 120 | **Protein:** 2 g | **Carbohydrates:** 20 g | **Dietary Fiber:** 5 g | **Sugars:** 8 g | **Fat:** 3 g | **Sodium:** 150 mg | **Potassium:** 400 mg | **Phosphorus:** 90 mg

Stir-Fried Tofu with Mixed Vegetables

Yield: 1 serving | **Prep time:** 10 minutes | **Cook time:** 10 minutes

INGREDIENTS:

- 1/2 cup firm tofu, pressed and cubed
- 1/2 tablespoon olive oil
- 1/4 cup sliced bell peppers (mix of red and yellow)
- 1/4 cup broccoli florets
- 1/4 cup sliced carrots
- 1/4 cup snap peas
- 1/2 garlic clove, minced
- 1 teaspoon low-sodium soy sauce
- 1/2 teaspoon sesame oil
- A pinch of black pepper

DIRECTIONS:

1. Heat the olive oil in a non-stick skillet over medium-high heat. Add the tofu cubes and fry until golden brown on all sides. Remove from the skillet and set aside.

2. Add garlic, bell peppers, broccoli, carrots, and snap peas in the same skillet. Stir-fry for about 5 minutes until the vegetables are tender but still crisp.

3. Return the tofu to the skillet. Add the low-sodium soy sauce, sesame oil, and black pepper. Stir well to combine and cook for an additional 2 minutes.

4. Taste and adjust the seasoning if necessary, considering the sodium content for a renal diet.

5. Serve hot.

NUTRITIONAL INFORMATION:

Calories: 250 | **Protein:** 12g | **Carbohydrates:** 18g | **Dietary Fiber:** 5g | **Sugars:** 6g | **Fat:** 16g | **Sodium:** 200mg | **Potassium:** 400mg | **Phosphorus:** 150mg

Herbed Chicken and Vegetable Skillet

Yield: 1 serving | **Prep time:** 10 minutes | **Cook time:** 20 minutes

INGREDIENTS:

- 1 (4 oz) chicken breast, cut into strips
- 1/2 tablespoon olive oil
- 1/4 teaspoon dried thyme
- 1/4 teaspoon dried rosemary
- 1/4 teaspoon dried oregano
- 1/4 cup carrots, sliced
- 1/4 cup zucchini, sliced
- 1/4 cup bell pepper, sliced
- 1/4 cup broccoli florets
- Salt substitute and black pepper to taste
- Fresh parsley, chopped for garnish

DIRECTIONS:

1. Heat olive oil in a large skillet over medium heat.

2. Season chicken strips with dried thyme, rosemary, oregano, salt substitute, and black pepper. Add to the skillet until browned and cooked, about 5-7 minutes per side. Remove chicken from the skillet and set aside.

3. Add the carrots, zucchini, bell pepper, and broccoli in the same skillet. Sauté for about 5-8 minutes or until vegetables are tender but crisp.

4. Return the cooked chicken to the skillet with the vegetables. Stir well to combine and heat through for another 2 minutes.

5. Adjust seasoning with salt substitute and black pepper if needed.

6. Garnish with fresh parsley before serving.

NUTRITIONAL INFORMATION:

Calories: 300 | **Protein:** 26 g | **Carbohydrates:** 15 g | **Dietary Fiber:** 4 g | **Sugars:** 5 g | **Fat:** 15 g | **Sodium:** 150 mg | **Potassium:** 600 mg | **Phosphorus:** 220 mg

Low-Phosphorus Cheese Pizza with Vegetables

Yield: 1 serving | **Prep time:** 15 minutes | **Cook time:** 20 minutes

INGREDIENTS:

- 1 small whole wheat pizza base (about 6-7 inches diameter)
- 1/4 cup low-phosphorus cheese (mozzarella-style, renal-friendly)
- 1/4 cup tomato sauce (low sodium)
- 1/4 cup bell peppers, thinly sliced
- 1/4 cup mushrooms, thinly sliced
- 1/4 cup red onion, thinly sliced
- 1 teaspoon olive oil
- A pinch of dried oregano
- A pinch of garlic powder
- Fresh basil leaves for garnish

DIRECTIONS:

1. Preheat your oven to 425°F (220°C).
2. Spread the tomato sauce evenly over the pizza base, leaving a small border around the edges.
3. Sprinkle the garlic powder and dried oregano over the tomato sauce.
4. Top the sauce with an even layer of sliced bell peppers, mushrooms, and red onion.
5. Sprinkle the low-phosphorus cheese over the top of the vegetables.
6. Drizzle olive oil lightly over the pizza.
7. Place the pizza on a baking tray and bake in the oven for 15-20 minutes, until the cheese is melted and bubbly and the crust is golden brown.
8. Remove from the oven and let cool for a few minutes. Garnish with fresh basil leaves before serving.

NUTRITIONAL INFORMATION:

Calories: 350 | **Protein:** 15 g | **Carbohydrates:** 45 g | **Dietary Fiber:** 5 g | **Sugars:** 8 g | **Fat:** 12 g | **Sodium:** 400 mg | **Potassium:** 300 mg | **Phosphorus:** 200 mg

Quinoa Salad with Roasted Vegetables

Yield: 1 serving | **Prep time:** 15 minutes | **Cook time:** 25 minutes

INGREDIENTS:

- 1/2 cup cooked quinoa
- 1/4 cup chopped zucchini
- 1/4 cup bell pepper strips
- 1/4 cup cherry tomatoes, halved
- 1/4 cup diced carrots
- 1 tablespoon olive oil
- Salt substitute and black pepper to taste
- 1 tablespoon lemon juice
- 1 teaspoon fresh parsley, chopped
- 1 teaspoon fresh basil, chopped

DIRECTIONS:

1. Preheat the oven to 400°F (200°C). Line a baking sheet with parchment paper.
2. Toss the zucchini, bell pepper, cherry tomatoes, and carrots with olive oil, salt substitute, and black pepper. Spread the vegetables evenly on the baking sheet.
3. Roast the vegetables in the oven for about 20-25 minutes, until tender and slightly caramelized, stirring halfway through the cooking time.
4. Combine the cooked quinoa and roasted vegetables in a large bowl. Add lemon juice and toss to mix well.
5. Stir in the chopped parsley and basil. Adjust the seasoning with more salt substitutes and black pepper if needed.
6. Serve the quinoa salad warm or at room temperature.

NUTRITIONAL INFORMATION:

Calories: 350 | **Protein:** 8 g | **Carbohydrates:** 45 g | **Dietary Fiber:** 7 g | **Sugars:** 5 g | **Fat:** 15 g | **Sodium:** 100 mg | **Potassium:** 500 mg | **Phosphorus:** 150 mg

Grilled Polenta with Roasted Vegetables

Yield: 1 serving | **Prep time:** 15 minutes | **Cook time:** 30 minutes

INGREDIENTS:

- 2 slices of pre-cooked polenta (about 1/2 inch thick)
- 1/4 cup zucchini, sliced
- 1/4 cup bell pepper, sliced
- 1/4 cup eggplant, sliced
- 1/4 cup cherry tomatoes
- 1/2 tablespoon olive oil
- A pinch of black pepper
- 1/2 teaspoon dried basil
- 1/2 teaspoon dried oregano

DIRECTIONS:

1. Preheat the oven to 425°F (220°C) for roasting the vegetables.
2. Toss the zucchini, bell pepper, eggplant, and cherry tomatoes with olive oil, black pepper, dried basil, and oregano. Spread them on a baking sheet in a single layer.
3. Roast the vegetables in the oven for about 20 minutes or until tender and slightly caramelized.
4. While roasting the vegetables, preheat the grill to medium heat. Grill the polenta slices on each side for 3-4 minutes until they have excellent grill marks.
5. Serve the grilled polenta topped with the roasted vegetables.

NUTRITIONAL INFORMATION:

Calories: 250 | **Protein:** 4g | **Carbohydrates:** 38g | **Dietary Fiber:** 5g | **Sugars:** 8g | **Fat:** 10g | **Sodium:** 150mg | **Potassium:** 525mg | **Phosphorus:** 100mg

Low-Sodium Beef Stroganoff

Yield: 1 serving | **Prep time:** 15 minutes | **Cook time:** 25 minutes

INGREDIENTS:

- 4 oz lean beef, sliced into thin strips
- 1/2 cup sliced mushrooms
- 1/4 cup diced onions
- 1 clove garlic, minced
- 1/2 tablespoon olive oil
- 1/2 cup low-sodium beef broth
- 1 tablespoon sour cream (low-fat, if preferred)
- 1 teaspoon all-purpose flour (for thickening, optional)
- A pinch of black pepper
- 1/2 cup cooked egg noodles (whole wheat, if preferred)
- Fresh parsley for garnish

DIRECTIONS:

1. Heat olive oil in a skillet over medium-high heat. Add the beef strips and cook until browned on all sides. Remove beef from the skillet and set aside.
2. In the same skillet, add the onions and garlic. Sauté until the onions are translucent.
3. Add the mushrooms to the skillet and cook until they are soft and their moisture has evaporated.
4. Return the beef to the skillet. Sprinkle with flour (if using) and stir to combine.
5. Pour in the low-sodium beef broth and bring to a simmer. Reduce heat and cook the mixture gently until the sauce thickens slightly for about 10 minutes.
6. Stir in the sour cream and a pinch of black pepper. Heat through, making sure not to boil, to avoid curdling the sour cream.
7. Serve the beef stroganoff over the cooked egg noodles, garnished with fresh parsley.

NUTRITIONAL INFORMATION:

Calories: 400 | **Protein:** 28 g | **Carbohydrates:** 30 g | **Dietary Fiber:** 3 g | **Sugars:** 4 g | **Fat:** 18 g | **Sodium:** 150 mg | **Potassium:** 650 mg | **Phosphorus:** 250 mg

Low-Sodium Chicken Tikka Masala

Yield: 1 serving | **Prep time:** 20 minutes | **Cook time:** 30 minutes

INGREDIENTS:

- 4 oz chicken breast, cut into cubes
- 1/2 cup plain, low-fat yogurt (for marinade)
- 1 teaspoon turmeric
- 1 teaspoon ground cumin
- 1 teaspoon ground coriander
- 1/2 teaspoon ground ginger
- 1/2 teaspoon garlic powder
- 1/2 tablespoon olive oil
- 1/4 cup diced onions
- 1/2 cup low-sodium canned tomatoes, crushed
- 1/4 cup coconut milk
- A pinch of garam masala
- Fresh cilantro for garnish

DIRECTIONS:

1. Mix yogurt with turmeric, cumin, coriander, ginger, and garlic powder in a bowl. Add the chicken cubes, ensuring they are well-coated with the marinade. Cover and refrigerate for at least 1 hour.

2. Heat olive oil in a skillet over medium heat. Add onions and sauté until they become translucent.

3. Add the marinated chicken to the skillet, discarding excess marinade. Cook until the chicken is browned on all sides.

4. Stir in the crushed tomatoes and simmer for 10 minutes, allowing the sauce to thicken slightly.

5. Add coconut milk and a pinch of garam masala, stirring well. Cook for 5-10 minutes until the chicken is fully cooked and the sauce has a creamy consistency.

6. Garnish with fresh cilantro before serving.

7. Serve with a side of steamed rice or a renal-friendly grain alternative.

NUTRITIONAL INFORMATION:

Calories: 350 | **Protein:** 28 g | **Carbohydrates:** 20 g | **Dietary Fiber:** 3 g | **Sugars:** 10 g | **Fat:** 18 g | **Sodium:** 200 mg | **Potassium:** 600 mg | **Phosphorus:** 250 mg

Low-Sodium Beef and Vegetable Kabobs

Yield: 1 serving | **Prep time:** 20 minutes | **Cook time:** 10 minutes

INGREDIENTS:

- 4 ounces beef sirloin, cut into 1-inch cubes
- 1/4 cup bell pepper, cut into 1-inch pieces
- 1/4 cup zucchini, sliced
- 1/4 cup cherry tomatoes
- 1/4 red onion, cut into wedges
- 1/2 tablespoon olive oil
- A pinch of black pepper
- 1/2 teaspoon dried oregano
- 1/2 teaspoon garlic powder

DIRECTIONS:

1. Preheat the grill to medium-high heat.

2. Thread the beef, bell peppers, zucchini, cherry tomatoes, and red onion onto skewers.

3. Mix the olive oil, black pepper, dried oregano, and garlic powder in a small bowl. Brush this mixture over the kabobs.

4. Place the kabobs on the grill and cook for about 10 minutes, turning occasionally, until the beef reaches the desired doneness and the vegetables are tender.

5. Serve the kabobs hot.

NUTRITIONAL INFORMATION:

Calories: 300 | **Protein:** 26g | **Carbohydrates:** 10g | **Dietary Fiber:** 2g | **Sugars:** 6g | **Fat:** 18g | **Sodium:** 75mg | **Potassium:** 650mg | **Phosphorus:** 250mg

Baked Haddock with Parsley Sauce

Yield: 1 serving | **Prep time:** 10 minutes | **Cook time:** 20 minutes

INGREDIENTS:

- 1 (6 oz) haddock fillet
- 1/2 tablespoon olive oil
- A pinch of black pepper
- For the Parsley Sauce:
- - 1/4 cup low-sodium chicken or vegetable broth
- - 1 teaspoon cornstarch
- - 1 tablespoon fresh parsley, finely chopped
- - 1 teaspoon lemon juice
- - A pinch of garlic powder

DIRECTIONS:

1. Preheat the oven to 375°F (190°C). Line a baking tray with parchment paper.
2. Place the haddock fillet on the prepared tray. Brush with olive oil and season with black pepper.
3. Bake in the oven for 15-20 minutes or until the fish flakes easily with a fork.
4. While the fish is baking, prepare the parsley sauce. In a small saucepan, whisk together the broth and cornstarch over medium heat until the cornstarch is dissolved.
5. Bring the mixture to a simmer, stirring constantly, until it thickens slightly. Stir in the parsley, lemon juice, and garlic powder. Remove from heat.
6. Transfer the haddock to a serving plate once it is cooked. Pour the parsley sauce over the haddock.
7. Serve immediately, garnished with additional fresh parsley if desired.

NUTRITIONAL INFORMATION:

Calories: 250 | **Protein:** 25 g | **Carbohydrates:** 4 g | **Dietary Fiber:** 0.5 g | **Sugars:** 0.5 g | **Fat:** 14 g | **Sodium:** 120 mg | **Potassium:** 600 mg | **Phosphorus:** 250 mg

Baked Trout with Dill and Lemon

Yield: 1 serving | **Prep time:** 10 minutes | **Cook time:** 15 minutes

INGREDIENTS:

- 1 (6 oz) trout fillet
- 1 tablespoon olive oil
- 1/2 lemon, thinly sliced
- 1 teaspoon fresh dill, chopped
- Salt substitute and black pepper to taste

DIRECTIONS:

1. Preheat your oven to 375°F (190°C). Line a baking sheet with parchment paper.
2. Place the trout fillet on the prepared baking sheet. Drizzle with olive oil and season with a salt substitute and black pepper.
3. Arrange the lemon slices on top of the trout fillet and sprinkle with chopped dill.
4. Bake in the preheated oven for about 12-15 minutes, or until the trout is cooked and flakes quickly with a fork.
5. Carefully remove the trout from the oven and transfer it to a serving plate.
6. Serve immediately, garnished with additional fresh dill if desired.

NUTRITIONAL INFORMATION:

Calories: 280 | **Protein:** 23 g | **Carbohydrates:** 0 g | **Dietary Fiber:** 0 g | **Sugars:** 0 g | **Fat:** 20 g | **Sodium:** 65 mg | **Potassium:** 500 mg | **Phosphorus:** 300 mg

Grilled Vegetable Skewers

Yield: 1 serving | **Prep time:** 15 minutes | **Cook time:** 10 minutes

INGREDIENTS:

- 1/2 zucchini, cut into 1/2-inch slices
- 1/2 yellow squash, cut into 1/2-inch slices
- 1/4 red bell pepper, cut into 1-inch pieces
- 1/4 green bell pepper, cut into 1-inch pieces
- 4 cherry tomatoes
- 1 tablespoon olive oil
- A pinch of dried oregano
- A pinch of black pepper
- Wooden or metal skewers (if using wooden skewers, soak in water for 30 minutes to prevent burning)

DIRECTIONS:

1. Preheat your grill to medium-high heat.
2. Thread the zucchini, yellow squash, bell peppers, and cherry tomatoes alternately onto the skewers.
3. Brush the vegetables lightly with olive oil and sprinkle with dried oregano and black pepper.
4. Place the skewers on the grill and cook for 4-5 minutes on each side or until the vegetables are tender and slightly charred.
5. Remove the skewers from the grill and let them cool for a few minutes before serving.
6. Enjoy your colorful and nutritious grilled vegetable skewers!

NUTRITIONAL INFORMATION:

Calories: 150 | **Protein:** 2 g | **Carbohydrates:** 12 g | **Dietary Fiber:** 3 g | **Sugars:** 6 g | **Fat:** 10 g | **Sodium:** 30 mg | **Potassium:** 500 mg | **Phosphorus:** 70 mg

Vegetable Lentil Stew

Yield: 1 serving | **Prep time:** 15 minutes | **Cook time:** 30 minutes

INGREDIENTS:

- 1/4 cup red lentils, rinsed
- 1 cup water
- 1/2 small carrot, diced
- 1/4 small onion, diced
- 1/2 stalk celery, diced
- 1/4 small red bell pepper, diced
- 1/2 garlic clove, minced
- 1/2 teaspoon olive oil
- 1/4 teaspoon dried thyme
- 1/4 teaspoon dried oregano
- A pinch of black pepper
- 1/2 cup low-sodium vegetable broth
- 1/2 tablespoon tomato paste
- 1/2 cup chopped spinach

DIRECTIONS:

1. Heat the olive oil over medium heat in a medium saucepan. Add the onion, garlic, carrot, celery, and red bell pepper. Sauté for 5 minutes until the vegetables start to soften.
2. Add the rinsed lentils, vegetable broth, water, tomato paste, thyme, oregano, and black pepper to the saucepan. Stir to combine.
3. Bring the mixture to a boil, then reduce the heat to low, cover, and simmer for 20-25 minutes or until the lentils are tender.
4. Stir in the chopped spinach and cook for 5 minutes or until the spinach is wilted.
5. Taste and adjust the seasoning if necessary, being mindful of the sodium content.

NUTRITIONAL INFORMATION:

Calories: 230 | **Protein:** 14g | **Carbohydrates:** 39g | **Dietary Fiber:** 15g | **Sugars:** 6g | **Fat:** 3g | **Sodium:** 200mg | **Potassium:** 600mg | **Phosphorus:** 200mg

Vegetable Paella

Yield: 1 serving | **Prep time:** 15 minutes | **Cook time:** 30 minutes

INGREDIENTS:

- 1/4 cup uncooked short-grain brown rice
- 1 cup low-sodium vegetable broth
- 1/4 cup diced bell peppers (a mix of colors)
- 1/4 cup diced tomatoes
- 1/4 cup artichoke hearts (canned in water, drained)
- 1/4 cup green peas (fresh or frozen and thawed)
- 1 tablespoon diced onion
- 1 clove garlic, minced
- 1/4 teaspoon smoked paprika
- A pinch of saffron threads (optional for flavor and color)
- 1 teaspoon olive oil
- Salt substitute and black pepper to taste
- Fresh parsley, chopped for garnish
- Lemon wedges for serving

DIRECTIONS:

1. Heat olive oil in a skillet over medium heat. Add onion and garlic, and sauté until translucent.
2. Stir in bell peppers and tomatoes, cooking until slightly softened.
3. Add the rice, smoked paprika, and saffron threads (if using) to the skillet. Stir until the rice is well coated with the spices.
4. Pour the low-sodium vegetable broth, simmer, then reduce heat to low. Cover and cook for about 20 minutes or until the rice is almost tender.
5. Add the artichoke hearts and peas to the skillet, gently folding them into the rice. Cover and cook for 10 minutes or until the rice is tender and the liquid is absorbed.
6. Remove from heat and let it sit, covered, for 5 minutes.
7. Season with salt substitute and black pepper to taste.
8. Serve the vegetable paella garnished with fresh parsley and lemon wedges on the side.

NUTRITIONAL INFORMATION:

Calories: 300 | **Protein:** 8 g | **Carbohydrates:** 50 g | **Dietary Fiber:** 8 g | **Sugars:** 5 g | **Fat:** 7 g | **Sodium:** 200 mg | **Potassium:** 400 mg | **Phosphorus:** 150 mg

Stuffed Peppers with Quinoa and Vegetables

Yield: 1 serving | **Prep time:** 15 minutes | **Cook time:** 30 minutes

INGREDIENTS:

- 1 large bell pepper, halved and seeds removed
- 1/2 cup cooked quinoa
- 1/4 cup finely chopped zucchini
- 1/4 cup finely chopped mushrooms
- 1/4 cup finely chopped carrots
- 1 tablespoon olive oil
- 1 clove garlic, minced
- 1 tablespoon low-sodium tomato sauce
- A pinch of dried oregano
- A pinch of dried basil
- Salt substitute and black pepper to taste
- Fresh parsley for garnish

DIRECTIONS:

1. Preheat your oven to 375°F (190°C).
2. In a skillet over medium heat, heat the olive oil and sauté garlic, zucchini, mushrooms, and carrots until they start to soften, about 5 minutes.
3. Stir in the cooked quinoa, tomato sauce, oregano, basil, salt substitute, and black pepper. Cook for an additional 2 minutes, then remove from heat.
4. Place the bell pepper halves in a baking dish and cut side up. Spoon the quinoa and vegetable mixture into each bell pepper half.
5. Cover the baking dish with aluminum foil and bake in the oven for about 20-25 minutes or until the peppers are tender.

6. Remove the foil and bake for 5 minutes to get a slightly crispy top.

7. Garnish with fresh parsley before serving.

NUTRITIONAL INFORMATION:

Calories: 320 | **Protein:** 9 g | **Carbohydrates:** 45 g | **Dietary Fiber:** 9 g | **Sugars:** 10 g | **Fat:** 12 g | **Sodium:** 100 mg | **Potassium:** 600 mg | **Phosphorus:** 200 mg

Kidney-Friendly Pasta Primavera

Yield: 1 serving | **Prep time:** 10 minutes | **Cook time:** 20 minutes

INGREDIENTS:

- 1 cup cooked whole wheat pasta (spaghetti or fettuccine)
- 1/4 cup sliced carrots
- 1/4 cup broccoli florets
- 1/4 cup sliced zucchini
- 1/4 cup red bell pepper strips
- 1 tablespoon olive oil
- 1 clove garlic, minced
- 1/4 cup low-sodium vegetable broth
- 1 teaspoon dried Italian herbs (basil, oregano, thyme)
- Salt substitute and black pepper to taste
- Fresh parsley, chopped for garnish
- 1 tablespoon grated Parmesan cheese (optional; ensure low-phosphorus if used)

DIRECTIONS:

1. Heat olive oil in a large skillet over medium heat. Add garlic and sauté for about 1 minute until fragrant.

2. Add carrots, broccoli, zucchini, and red bell pepper to the skillet. Stir-fry for about 5 minutes until vegetables are just tender.

3. Pour the low-sodium vegetable broth and add the dried Italian herbs. Stir well to combine—season with salt substitute and black pepper to taste. Simmer for 5-7 minutes until the vegetables are fully cooked and the broth slightly reduces.

4. Toss the cooked pasta into the skillet with the vegetables and mix well to ensure the pasta is evenly coated with the sauce and vegetables.

5. Cook together for 2 minutes, then remove from heat.

6. If desired, Serve the pasta primavera garnished with fresh parsley and a sprinkle of grated Parmesan cheese.

NUTRITIONAL INFORMATION:

Calories: 320 | **Protein:** 10 g | **Carbohydrates:** 45 g | **Dietary Fiber:** 8 g | **Sugars:** 5 g | **Fat:** 12 g | **Sodium:** 150 mg | **Potassium:** 350 mg | **Phosphorus:** 100 mg

Baked Chicken with Thyme and Vegetables

Yield: 1 serving | **Prep time:** 15 minutes | **Cook time:** 25 minutes

INGREDIENTS:

- 1 (6 oz) skinless chicken breast
- 1/2 cup carrots, sliced
- 1/2 cup zucchini, sliced
- 1/2 cup bell peppers, sliced
- 1 tablespoon olive oil
- 1/2 teaspoon dried thyme
- A pinch of black pepper
- A pinch of garlic powder

DIRECTIONS:

1. Preheat your oven to 375°F (190°C). Line a baking sheet with parchment paper.
2. In a bowl, toss the sliced carrots, zucchini, and bell peppers with half the olive oil, a pinch of black pepper, and garlic powder.
3. Place the vegetables on one side of the prepared baking sheet.
4. Place the chicken breast on the other side of the baking sheet. Brush the chicken with olive oil and sprinkle with dried thyme and black pepper.
5. Bake in the preheated oven for 20-25 minutes, or until the chicken is cooked through (reaching an internal temperature of 165°F) and the vegetables are tender.
6. Remove from the oven and let it rest for a few minutes before serving.
7. Serve the baked chicken with the roasted thyme vegetables on the side.

NUTRITIONAL INFORMATION:

Calories: 350 | **Protein:** 36 g | **Carbohydrates:** 15 g | **Dietary Fiber:** 4 g | **Sugars:** 6 g | **Fat:** 16 g | **Sodium:** 120 mg | **Potassium:** 800 mg | **Phosphorus:** 300 mg

Grilled Lemon-Herb Chicken Breast

Yield: 1 serving | **Prep time:** 10 minutes | **Cook time:** 15 minutes

INGREDIENTS:

- 1 boneless, skinless chicken breast (about 6 oz)
- Juice of 1/2 lemon
- 1 teaspoon olive oil
- 1 clove garlic, minced
- A pinch of dried rosemary
- A pinch of dried thyme
- A pinch of black pepper

DIRECTIONS:

1. Mix the lemon juice, olive oil, minced garlic, rosemary, thyme, and black pepper in a small bowl.
2. Place the chicken breast in a shallow dish and pour the lemon-herb mixture. Make sure the chicken is well coated. Marinate it in the refrigerator for at least 30 minutes.
3. Preheat the grill to medium-high heat.
4. Remove the chicken from the marinade, letting excess drip off. Place the chicken on the grill.
5. Grill the chicken for 7-8 minutes per side or until the internal temperature reaches 165°F (74°C) and the juices run clear.
6. Remove the chicken from the grill and let it rest for a few minutes before serving.
7. Serve the grilled chicken with a wedge of lemon.

NUTRITIONAL INFORMATION:

Calories: 220 | **Protein:** 35 g | **Carbohydrates:** 1 g | **Dietary Fiber:** 0 g | **Sugars:** 0 g | **Fat:** 9 g | **Sodium:** 70 mg | **Potassium:** 370 mg | **Phosphorus:** 290 mg

CHAPTER 8

Snacks &
Side Dishes

—

Cauliflower Buffalo Bites

Yield: 1 serving | **Prep time:** 10 minutes | **Cook time:** 25 minutes

INGREDIENTS:

- 1 cup cauliflower florets
- 1 tablespoon olive oil
- 2 tablespoons hot sauce (low sodium)
- 1/2 teaspoon garlic powder
- 1/2 teaspoon paprika
- Black pepper to taste

DIRECTIONS:

1. Preheat your oven to 425°F (220°C). Line a baking sheet with parchment paper.

2. Combine the olive oil, hot sauce, garlic powder, paprika, and black pepper in a large bowl. Mix well.

3. Add the cauliflower florets to the bowl and toss until they are fully coated with the sauce mixture.

4. Spread the coated cauliflower florets in a single layer on the prepared baking sheet.

5. Bake in the preheated oven for about 20-25 minutes or until the cauliflower is tender and beginning to brown.

6. Remove from the oven and let cool slightly before serving.

NUTRITIONAL INFORMATION:

Calories: 150 | **Protein:** 3g | **Carbohydrates:** 11g | **Dietary Fiber:** 4g | **Sugars:** 4g | **Fat:** 11g | **Sodium:** 200mg | **Potassium:** 450mg | **Phosphorus:** 70mg

Apple Slices with Almond Butter

Yield: 1 serving | **Prep time:** 5 minutes | **Cook time:** 0 minutes

INGREDIENTS:

- 1 medium apple, cored and sliced
- 2 tablespoons almond butter

DIRECTIONS:

1. Core the apple and cut it into slices.
2. Spread almond butter evenly over the apple slices.

NUTRITIONAL INFORMATION:

Calories: 280 | **Protein:** 5g | **Carbohydrates:** 34g | **Dietary Fiber:** 6g | **Sugars:** 25g | **Fat:** 16g | **Sodium:** 0mg | **Potassium:** 400mg | **Phosphorus:** 100mg

Low-Sodium Cheese Cubes

Yield: 1 serving | **Prep time:** 5 minutes | **Cook time:** 0 minutes

INGREDIENTS:

- 2 ounces low-sodium cheese (choose varieties like Swiss, mozzarella, or ricotta, which typically have lower sodium content)

DIRECTIONS:

1. Select a block of low-sodium cheese from the varieties recommended.
2. Using a knife, carefully cut the cheese into 1-inch cubes.
3. Place the cheese cubes on a plate and serve immediately. Alternatively, refrigerate them in an airtight container for a later snack.

NUTRITIONAL INFORMATION:

Calories: 200 | **Protein:** 14g | **Carbohydrates:** 2g | **Dietary Fiber:** 0g | **Sugars:** 1g | **Fat:** 15g | **Sodium:** 60mg | **Potassium:** 20mg | **Phosphorus:** 100mg

Pear and Cheese Slices

Yield: 1 serving | **Prep time:** 5 minutes | **Cook time:** 0 minutes

INGREDIENTS:

- 1 medium pear
- 2 slices of low-sodium cheese (such as Swiss or mozzarella)

DIRECTIONS:

1. Wash the pear and cut it into thin slices, removing the core.
2. Cut the low-sodium cheese into thin slices.
3. Alternate layers of pear and cheese slices on a plate or arrange them in a pattern of your choice.
4. Serve immediately for a fresh, sweet, and savory snack.

NUTRITIONAL INFORMATION:

Calories: 200 | **Protein:** 10g | **Carbohydrates:** 25g | **Dietary Fiber:** 5g | **Sugars:** 17g | **Fat:** 8g | **Sodium:** 120mg | **Potassium:** 200mg | **Phosphorus:** 150mg

Cucumber Slices with Low-Sodium Hummus

Yield: 1 serving | **Prep time:** 10 minutes | **Cook time:** 0 minutes

INGREDIENTS:

- 1 medium cucumber, sliced
- 1/4 cup low-sodium hummus

DIRECTIONS:

1. Wash the cucumber thoroughly and slice it into thin rounds.
2. Spoon the low-sodium hummus into a small bowl.
3. Arrange the cucumber slices around the bowl of hummus on a plate for dipping.
4. Enjoy the cucumber slices by dipping them into the hummus.

NUTRITIONAL INFORMATION:

Calories: 150 | **Protein:** 5g | **Carbohydrates:** 20g | **Dietary Fiber:** 4g | **Sugars:** 5g | **Fat:** 7g | **Sodium:** 200mg | **Potassium:** 360mg | **Phosphorus:** 120mg

Pineapple and Cottage Cheese

Yield: 1 serving | **Prep time:** 5 minutes | **Cook time:** 0 minutes

INGREDIENTS:

- 1/2 cup low-fat cottage cheese
- 1/2 cup fresh pineapple chunks

DIRECTIONS:

1. Place the low-fat cottage cheese in a serving bowl.
2. Top the cottage cheese with fresh pineapple chunks.
3. Serve immediately or chill in the refrigerator for a refreshing and cool snack.

NUTRITIONAL INFORMATION:

Calories: 150 | **Protein:** 14g | **Carbohydrates:** 20g | **Dietary Fiber:** 1g | **Sugars:** 15g | **Fat:** 2g | **Sodium:** 400mg | **Potassium:** 200mg | **Phosphorus:** 120mg

Melon Balls (Cantaloupe or Honeydew)

Yield: 1 serving | **Prep time:** 10 minutes | **Cook time:** 0 minutes

INGREDIENTS:

- 1 cup melon balls (from either cantaloupe or honeydew)

DIRECTIONS:

1. Cut the melon in half and remove the seeds.
2. Using a melon baller, scoop out balls of melon flesh from either the cantaloupe or honeydew.
3. Place the melon balls into a serving bowl or store them in an airtight container in the refrigerator until ready to serve.
4. Enjoy as a refreshing snack or dessert.

NUTRITIONAL INFORMATION:

Calories: 60 | **Protein:** 1g | **Carbohydrates:** 14g | **Dietary Fiber:** 1g | **Sugars:** 13g | **Fat:** 0g | **Sodium:** 30mg | **Potassium:** 427mg | **Phosphorus:** 26mg

Carrot Sticks with Low-Phosphorus Ranch Dip

Yield: 1 serving | **Prep time:** 10 minutes | **Cook time:** 0 minutes

INGREDIENTS:

- 1/2 cup carrot sticks
- 2 tablespoons homemade low-phosphorus ranch dip

For Low-Phosphorus Ranch Dip:

- 1/4 cup mayonnaise
- 1/4 cup sour cream (low-phosphorus alternative)
- 1 teaspoon dried dill
- 1/2 teaspoon garlic powder
- 1/2 teaspoon onion powder
- A pinch of black pepper
- 1 teaspoon lemon juice

DIRECTIONS:

1. Prepare the ranch dip by mixing mayonnaise, sour cream, dried dill, garlic powder, onion powder, black pepper, and lemon juice in a small bowl until well combined.

2. Cut carrots into sticks, if not pre-cut.

3. Serve carrot sticks alongside the homemade low-phosphorus ranch dip for dipping.

NUTRITIONAL INFORMATION:

Calories: 220 | **Protein:** 2g | **Carbohydrates:** 10g | **Dietary Fiber:** 2g | **Sugars:** 5g | **Fat:** 20g | **Sodium:** 200mg | **Potassium:** 200mg | **Phosphorus:** 50mg

Bell Pepper Strips with Guacamole

Yield: 1 serving | **Prep time:** 10 minutes | **Cook time:** 0 minutes

INGREDIENTS:

- 1/2 large red bell pepper
- 1/2 large yellow bell pepper
- 1/4 cup homemade guacamole

For Homemade Guacamole:

- 1/2 ripe avocado
- 1 tablespoon diced tomato
- 1 tablespoon finely chopped onion
- 1 teaspoon lime juice
- A pinch of black pepper

DIRECTIONS:

1. Rinse the bell peppers under cold water. Pat dry and then cut into strips.

2. Prepare the guacamole by mashing the avocado in a small bowl until it reaches your desired consistency.

3. Mix the diced tomato, chopped onion, lime juice, and a pinch of black pepper into the mashed avocado.

4. Serve the bell pepper strips alongside the freshly made guacamole for dipping.

NUTRITIONAL INFORMATION:

Calories: 180 | **Protein:** 3g | **Carbohydrates:** 20g | **Dietary Fiber:** 7g | **Sugars:** 8g | **Fat:** 12g | **Sodium:** 20mg | **Potassium:** 650mg | **Phosphorus:** 75mg

Boiled Egg Whites

Yield: 1 serving | **Prep time:** 2 minutes | **Cook time:** 10 minutes

INGREDIENTS:
- 2 large eggs

DIRECTIONS:

1. Cover the eggs in a small saucepan with cold water by 1 inch.
2. Bring the water to a boil over high heat. Once boiling, cover the saucepan and remove it from the heat.
3. Let the eggs stand in the hot water for 9 minutes for firm egg whites.
4. After 9 minutes, transfer the eggs to a bowl of ice water to cool down for about 3 minutes.
5. Peel the eggs and slice them in half. Remove the yolks and use the egg whites as desired.

NUTRITIONAL INFORMATION:

Calories: 34 | **Protein:** 7g | **Carbohydrates:** 0.5g | **Dietary Fiber:** 0g | **Sugars:** 0.5g | **Fat:** 0.1g | **Sodium:** 110mg | **Potassium:** 108mg | **Phosphorus:** 10mg

Fresh Berry Salad

Yield: 1 serving | **Prep time:** 10 minutes | **Cook time:** 0 minutes

INGREDIENTS:
- 1/2 cup strawberries, sliced
- 1/2 cup blueberries
- 1/2 cup raspberries
- 1 tablespoon chopped fresh mint
- 1 teaspoon honey (optional)
- A squeeze of fresh lemon juice (optional)

DIRECTIONS:

1. In a mixing bowl, gently combine the sliced strawberries, blueberries, and raspberries.
2. If using, drizzle the honey over the berries for a touch of sweetness.
3. Add a squeeze of fresh lemon juice to brighten the flavors.
4. Sprinkle chopped fresh mint over the salad for an aromatic freshness.
5. Toss everything gently to combine without breaking the berries.
6. Serve immediately to enjoy the freshness of the berries.

NUTRITIONAL INFORMATION:

Calories: 120 | **Protein:** 2g | **Carbohydrates:** 29g | **Dietary Fiber:** 8g | **Sugars:** 17g | **Fat:** 0.5g | **Sodium:** 5mg | **Potassium:** 200mg | **Phosphorus:** 35mg

Roasted Chickpeas
(Low-Sodium)

Yield: 1 serving | **Prep time:** 5 minutes | **Cook time:** 40 minutes

INGREDIENTS:

- 1/2 cup canned chickpeas, rinsed and drained
- 1/2 tablespoon olive oil
- A pinch of black pepper
- 1/4 teaspoon garlic powder
- 1/4 teaspoon smoked paprika (optional)

DIRECTIONS:

1. Preheat your oven to 400°F (200°C). Line a baking sheet with parchment paper.
2. Rinse the chickpeas under cold water and drain them. Pat dry with a kitchen towel to remove as much moisture as possible.
3. toss the chickpeas with olive oil, black pepper, garlic powder, and smoked paprika until evenly coated.
4. Spread the chickpeas in a single layer on the prepared baking sheet.
5. Roast in the oven for 35-40 minutes or until crispy and golden. Shake the pan or stir the chickpeas halfway through to ensure even roasting.
6. Let them cool before serving to enhance their crispiness.

NUTRITIONAL INFORMATION:

Calories: 150 | **Protein:** 5g | **Carbohydrates:** 20g | **Dietary Fiber:** 6g | **Sugars:** 3g | **Fat:** 7g | **Sodium:** 15mg | **Potassium:** 200mg | **Phosphorus:** 120mg

Sliced Peaches with Cottage Cheese

Yield: 1 serving | **Prep time:** 5 minutes | **Cook time:** 0 minutes

INGREDIENTS:

- 1/2 cup sliced fresh peaches
- 1/2 cup low-fat cottage cheese

DIRECTIONS:

1. Rinse the fresh peaches under cold water. Pat dry with a kitchen towel.
2. Slice the peaches into thin slices, removing the pit.
3. Place the sliced peaches in a serving bowl.
4. Top the sliced peaches with the low-fat cottage cheese.
5. Serve immediately or chill in the refrigerator for a refreshing snack.

NUTRITIONAL INFORMATION:

Calories: 120 | **Protein:** 14g | **Carbohydrates:** 13g | **Dietary Fiber:** 1g | **Sugars:** 12g | **Fat:** 2.5g | **Sodium:** 350mg | **Potassium:** 200mg | **Phosphorus:** 100mg

Steamed Edamame

(Lightly Salted)

Yield: 1 serving | **Prep time:** 5 minutes | **Cook time:** 5 minutes

INGREDIENTS:

- 1/2 cup frozen edamame (in pods)
- A pinch of salt (optional; adjust according to dietary restrictions)

DIRECTIONS:

1. Bring a pot of water to a boil. Add a steamer basket to the pot.
2. Place the frozen edamame in the steamer basket. Cover the pot with a lid.
3. Steam the edamame for about 5 minutes or until they are thoroughly heated through and tender.
4. Remove the edamame from the steamer and sprinkle with a pinch of salt, if desired. Be cautious with the amount of salt if you're on a low-sodium diet.
5. Serve the edamame warm, and enjoy by squeezing the beans out of the pods directly into your mouth.

NUTRITIONAL INFORMATION:

Calories: 100 | **Protein:** 8g | **Carbohydrates:** 9g | **Dietary Fiber:** 4g | **Sugars:** 2g | **Fat:** 4g | **Sodium:** 15mg (without added salt) | **Potassium:** 200mg | **Phosphorus:** 100mg

Greek Yogurt with Honey and Berries

Yield: 1 serving | **Prep time:** 5 minutes | **Cook time:** 0 minutes

INGREDIENTS:

- 3/4 cup non-fat Greek yogurt
- 1 tablespoon honey
- 1/2 cup mixed berries (such as strawberries, blueberries, and raspberries)

DIRECTIONS:

1. Place the Greek yogurt in a serving bowl.
2. Drizzle the honey over the yogurt.
3. Rinse the mixed berries and gently pat them dry. If using strawberries, slice them into halves or quarters, depending on their size.
4. Top the yogurt with the mixed berries.
5. Serve immediately for a refreshing and nutritious snack or dessert.

NUTRITIONAL INFORMATION:

Calories: 180 | **Protein:** 19g | **Carbohydrates:** 30g | **Dietary Fiber:** 2g | **Sugars:** 27g | **Fat:** 0g | **Sodium:** 60mg | **Potassium:** 240mg | **Phosphorus:** 150mg

Air-Popped Popcorn
(Unsalted)

Yield: 1 serving | **Prep time:** 2 minutes | **Cook time:** 3 minutes

INGREDIENTS:

- 1/4 cup popcorn kernels (for air popping)

DIRECTIONS:

1. Measure 1/4 cup of popcorn kernels.
2. Place the kernels in an air popper machine.
3. Turn on the machine and pop the kernels until the popping slows to several seconds between pops.
4. Once popping is complete, turn off the machine and carefully remove the popcorn from a serving bowl.
5. Serve the popcorn unsalted or add a renal diet-friendly seasoning, such as a small amount of nutritional yeast or a salt-free seasoning blend for extra flavor.

NUTRITIONAL INFORMATION:

Calories: 90 | **Protein:** 3g | **Carbohydrates:** 18g | **Dietary Fiber:** 4g | **Sugars:** 0g | **Fat:** 1g | **Sodium:** 0mg | **Potassium:** 75mg | **Phosphorus:** 100mg

Grilled Zucchini Slices

Yield: 1 serving | **Prep time:** 5 minutes | **Cook time:** 10 minutes

INGREDIENTS:

- 1 medium zucchini
- 1/2 tablespoon olive oil
- A pinch of black pepper
- A pinch of garlic powder (optional)

DIRECTIONS:

1. Preheat the grill to medium-high heat.
2. Slice the zucchini into 1/4-inch thick rounds.
3. toss the zucchini slices with olive oil, black pepper, and garlic powder until evenly coated.
4. Place the zucchini slices on the grill and cook for 4-5 minutes on each side until tender and grill marks appear.
5. Remove from the grill and serve immediately.

NUTRITIONAL INFORMATION:

Calories: 80 | **Protein:** 2g | **Carbohydrates:** 6g | **Dietary Fiber:** 2g | **Sugars:** 4g | **Fat:** 6g | **Sodium:** 10mg | **Potassium:** 512mg | **Phosphorus:** 58mg

Baked Kale Chips

Yield: 1 serving | **Prep time:** 5 minutes | **Cook time:** 10 minutes

INGREDIENTS:

- 1 cup kale leaves, washed, dried, and torn into bite-sized pieces
- 1/2 tablespoon olive oil
- A pinch of salt (optional; consider using a minimal amount or none for a low-sodium diet)

DIRECTIONS:

1. Preheat the oven to 350°F (175°C).
2. In a bowl, toss the kale leaves with olive oil until evenly coated. If using, lightly sprinkle with a pinch of salt.
3. Arrange the kale pieces in a single layer on a baking sheet lined with parchment paper.
4. Bake in the oven for 10 minutes or until the edges are slightly brown but not burnt.
5. Let the kale chips cool for a few minutes before serving; they will become crisper as they cool.

NUTRITIONAL INFORMATION:

Calories: 80 | **Protein:** 2g | **Carbohydrates:** 8g | **Dietary Fiber:** 1.5g | **Sugars:** 0g | **Fat:** 5g | **Sodium:** 25mg (without added salt) | **Potassium:** 299mg | **Phosphorus:** 36mg

Sugar Snap Peas with Creamy Dip

Yield: 1 serving | **Prep time:** 10 minutes | **Cook time:** 0 minutes

INGREDIENTS:

- 1/2 cup sugar snap peas, washed and trimmed
- 2 tablespoons low-fat Greek yogurt
- 1 tablespoon mayonnaise (low sodium)
- 1/2 teaspoon dried dill
- A pinch of garlic powder
- A pinch of black pepper

DIRECTIONS:

1. In a small bowl, mix the Greek yogurt, mayonnaise, dried dill, garlic powder, and black pepper until well combined to make the creamy dip.
2. Place the washed and trimmed sugar snap peas on a plate.
3. Serve the sugar snap peas with the bowl of creamy dip on the side for dipping.

NUTRITIONAL INFORMATION:

Calories: 100 | **Protein:** 3g | **Carbohydrates:** 8g | **Dietary Fiber:** 2g | **Sugars:** 4g | **Fat:** 6g | **Sodium:** 70mg | **Potassium:** 150mg | **Phosphorus:** 60mg

Homemade Low-Sodium Salsa with Baked Tortilla Chips

Yield: 1 serving | **Prep time:** 15 minutes | **Cook time:** 10 minutes

INGREDIENTS:

For the Salsa:
- 1/2 cup diced tomatoes
- 1 tablespoon diced red onion
- 1 tablespoon chopped fresh cilantro
- 1/2 small jalapeño, seeded and minced (optional)
- 1 teaspoon lime juice
- A pinch of black pepper

For the Baked Tortilla Chips:
- 1 corn tortilla
- 1/2 teaspoon olive oil
- A pinch of chili powder (optional)

DIRECTIONS:

1. Make the Salsa: In a small bowl, combine diced tomatoes, red onion, cilantro, jalapeño (if using), lime juice, and black pepper. Mix well and set aside to allow the flavors to meld.

2. Prepare the Tortilla Chips: Preheat your oven to 350°F (175°C). Brush both sides of the corn tortilla with olive oil and lightly sprinkle with chili powder if desired. Cut the tortilla into six wedges.

3. Place the tortilla wedges on a baking sheet in a single layer and bake in the oven for 10 minutes or until crisp and lightly golden.

4. Serve: Enjoy the baked tortilla chips with the homemade low-sodium salsa.

NUTRITIONAL INFORMATION:

Calories: 150 | **Protein:** 3g | **Carbohydrates:** 23g | **Dietary Fiber:** 4g | **Sugars:** 4g | **Fat:** 6g | **Sodium:** 60mg | **Potassium:** 300mg | **Phosphorus:** 60mg

Rice Cakes Topped with Avocado

Yield: 1 serving | **Prep time:** 5 minutes | **Cook time:** 0 minutes

INGREDIENTS:
- 2 plain rice cakes
- 1/2 ripe avocado
- A pinch of black pepper
- A squeeze of lemon juice (optional)

DIRECTIONS:

1. Mash the half avocado in a small bowl until it reaches a smooth consistency.

2. Mix a squeeze of lemon juice with the mashed avocado. The lemon juice adds flavor and helps prevent the avocado from browning.

3. Spread the mashed avocado evenly over the two rice cakes.

4. Season with a pinch of black pepper to taste.

5. Serve immediately for the best texture and flavor.

NUTRITIONAL INFORMATION:

Calories: 200 | **Protein:** 3g | **Carbohydrates:** 27g | **Dietary Fiber:** 7g | **Sugars:** 1g | **Fat:** 10g | **Sodium:** 20mg | **Potassium:** 500mg | **Phosphorus:** 60mg

Chilled Gazpacho Soup

Yield: 1 serving | **Prep time:** 15 minutes | **Cook time:** 0 minutes (requires chilling)

INGREDIENTS:

- 1/2 cup cucumber, peeled and diced
- 1/2 cup tomato, diced
- 1/4 cup red bell pepper, diced
- 1/4 cup green bell pepper, diced
- 1 tablespoon red onion, diced
- 1/2 garlic clove, minced
- 1/2 cup low-sodium vegetable broth
- 1 teaspoon olive oil
- 1 tablespoon lime juice
- A pinch of black pepper
- A pinch of cumin (optional)
- Fresh cilantro for garnish (optional)

DIRECTIONS:

1. In a blender, combine cucumber, tomato, red and green bell peppers, red onion, garlic, low-sodium vegetable broth, olive oil, lime juice, black pepper, and cumin if using. Blend until smooth.
2. Taste and adjust the seasoning, adding more lime juice or pepper if desired.
3. Chill the soup in the refrigerator for at least 1 hour or until cold.
4. Serve the chilled gazpacho garnished with fresh cilantro, if desired.

NUTRITIONAL INFORMATION:

Calories: 100 | **Protein:** 2g | **Carbohydrates:** 14g | **Dietary Fiber:** 3g | **Sugars:** 8g | **Fat:** 5g | **Sodium:** 50mg | **Potassium:** 350mg | **Phosphorus:** 60mg

Steamed Broccoli Florets

Yield: 1 serving | **Prep time:** 5 minutes | **Cook time:** 5 minutes

INGREDIENTS:

- 1 cup fresh broccoli florets

DIRECTIONS:

1. Wash the broccoli florets under cold water.
2. Fill a pot with an inch of water and bring it to a boil. Place a steamer basket in the pot, ensuring the water does not touch the bottom of the basket.
3. Add the broccoli florets to the steamer basket. Cover the pot with a lid.
4. Steam the broccoli over medium heat for about 5 minutes or until the florets are tender but still bright green.
5. Remove the broccoli from the steamer and serve immediately.

NUTRITIONAL INFORMATION:

Calories: 55 | **Protein:** 3.7g | **Carbohydrates:** 11g | **Dietary Fiber:** 5.1g | **Sugars:** 2.6g | **Fat:** 0.6g | **Sodium:** 50mg | **Potassium:** 460mg | **Phosphorus:** 105mg

Oven-Baked Sweet Potato Fries

Yield: 1 serving | **Prep time:** 10 minutes | **Cook time:** 25 minutes

INGREDIENTS:

- 1 medium sweet potato
- 1/2 tablespoon olive oil
- A pinch of black pepper
- A pinch of garlic powder (optional)

DIRECTIONS:

1. Preheat the oven to 425°F (220°C). Line a baking sheet with parchment paper.
2. Peel the sweet potato and cut it into 1/4-inch thick fries.
3. toss the sweet potato fries with olive oil, black pepper, and garlic powder until evenly coated.
4. Spread the fries in a single layer on the prepared baking sheet, ensuring they do not touch too much to allow for even cooking.
5. Bake in the preheated oven for 25 minutes or until tender and lightly browned, turning once halfway through the cooking time.
6. Serve the sweet potato fries immediately.

NUTRITIONAL INFORMATION:

Calories: 200 | **Protein:** 2g | **Carbohydrates:** 26g | **Dietary Fiber:** 4g | **Sugars:** 5g | **Fat:** 10g | **Sodium:** 70mg | **Potassium:** 440mg | **Phosphorus:** 60mg

Low-Sodium Pickles

Yield: 1 serving | **Prep time:** 10 minutes | **Cook time:** 0 minutes

(requires at least 24 hours for pickling)

INGREDIENTS:

- 1/2 cup cucumber slices
- 1/2 cup white vinegar
- 1/2 cup water
- 1 tablespoon sugar
- 1/2 teaspoon mustard seeds
- 1/4 teaspoon whole black peppercorns
- 1 clove garlic, peeled and lightly crushed
- 1 sprig of fresh dill

DIRECTIONS:

1. Combine the vinegar, water, and sugar in a saucepan. Heat over medium heat, stirring until the sugar dissolves.
2. layer the cucumber slices, mustard seeds, black peppercorns, garlic, and dill in a clean jar.
3. Pour the hot vinegar mixture over the cucumbers in the jar, ensuring the cucumbers are fully submerged.
4. Let the jar cool to room temperature, then seal with a lid.
5. Refrigerate the pickles for at least 24 hours to allow the flavors to develop. The pickles will be kept in the refrigerator for up to 2 weeks.

NUTRITIONAL INFORMATION:

Calories: 50 | **Protein:** 1g | **Carbohydrates:** 12g | **Dietary Fiber:** 1g | **Sugars:** 10g | **Fat:** 0g | **Sodium:** 10mg | **Potassium:** 75mg | **Phosphorus:** 10mg

Homemade Low-Sodium Pesto with Whole Wheat Crackers

Yield: 1 serving | **Prep time:** 10 minutes | **Cook time:** 0 minutes

INGREDIENTS:

For the Low-Sodium Pesto:
- 1/2 cup fresh basil leaves
- 1 tablespoon pine nuts
- 1 garlic clove
- 2 tablespoons grated Parmesan cheese (low-sodium variety)
- 2 tablespoons olive oil
- Black pepper, to taste

For Serving:
- 10 whole wheat crackers

DIRECTIONS:

1. Combine the fresh basil leaves, pine nuts, and garlic in a food processor or blender. Pulse until coarsely chopped.

2. Add the grated Parmesan cheese and olive oil to the basil mixture. Blend until smooth, scraping down the sides as necessary — season with black pepper to taste.

3. Transfer the pesto to a small bowl.

4. Serve the homemade low-sodium pesto with whole wheat crackers on the side for dipping or spreading.

NUTRITIONAL INFORMATION:

Calories: 350 | **Protein:** 10g | **Carbohydrates:** 24g | **Dietary Fiber:** 4g | **Sugars:** 2g | **Fat:** 25g | **Sodium:** 200mg | **Potassium:** 150mg | **Phosphorus:** 100mg

Low-Phosphorus Macaroni Salad

Yield: 1 serving | **Prep time:** 15 minutes | **Cook time:** 10 minutes

INGREDIENTS:

- 1/2 cup low-phosphorus macaroni pasta (cooked according to package instructions and cooled)
- 1/4 cup diced celery
- 1/4 cup diced red bell pepper
- 1 tablespoon chopped red onion
- 2 tablespoons mayonnaise (low sodium)
- 1 teaspoon white vinegar
- A pinch of black pepper
- A pinch of dried dill (optional)

DIRECTIONS:

1. In a large bowl, combine the cooked and cooled macaroni with the diced celery, red bell pepper, and chopped red onion.

2. Mix the mayonnaise, white vinegar, black pepper, and dried dill in a small bowl until well combined.

3. Pour the dressing over the macaroni mixture and stir until evenly coated.

4. Cover and refrigerate the salad for at least 1 hour to allow the flavors to meld.

5. Serve the macaroni salad chilled.

NUTRITIONAL INFORMATION:

Calories: 320 | **Protein:** 7g | **Carbohydrates:** 37g | **Dietary Fiber:** 2g | **Sugars:** 3g | **Fat:** 16g | **Sodium:** 150mg | **Potassium:** 200mg | **Phosphorus:** 100mg

Roasted Brussels Sprouts

Yield: 1 serving | **Prep time:** 10 minutes | **Cook time:** 20 minutes

INGREDIENTS:

- 1 cup Brussels sprouts, halved
- 1 teaspoon olive oil
- A pinch of black pepper
- A pinch of garlic powder (optional)

DIRECTIONS:

1. Preheat your oven to 400°F (200°C).
2. Wash the Brussels sprouts and cut them in half.
3. toss the Brussels sprouts with olive oil, black pepper, and garlic powder until evenly coated.
4. Spread the Brussels sprouts on a baking sheet in a single layer and cut side down.
5. Roast in the preheated oven for about 20 minutes or until they are tender and the edges start to crisp and brown.
6. Remove from the oven and serve immediately.

NUTRITIONAL INFORMATION:

Calories: 100 | **Protein:** 4g | **Carbohydrates:** 14g | **Dietary Fiber:** 6g | **Sugars:** 3g | **Fat:** 4g | **Sodium:** 30mg | **Potassium:** 450mg | **Phosphorus:** 100mg

Low-Sodium Deviled Eggs

Yield: 1 serving (makes 4 halves) | **Prep time:** 10 minutes | **Cook time:** 10 minutes

INGREDIENTS:

- 2 large eggs
- 1 tablespoon low-fat mayonnaise
- 1/2 teaspoon Dijon mustard
- A pinch of black pepper
- A pinch of paprika (for garnish)
- Fresh chives, chopped (for garnish, optional)

DIRECTIONS:

1. Place the eggs in a saucepan and cover them with water. Bring to a boil, then cover, remove from heat, and let sit for 9 minutes.
2. After 9 minutes, place eggs in cold water to cool, then peel them.
3. Cut the eggs in half lengthwise. Remove the yolks and place them in a bowl.
4. Mash the yolks with a fork and mix in the low-fat mayonnaise, Dijon mustard, and black pepper until smooth.
5. Spoon or pipe the yolk mixture back into the egg whites.
6. Sprinkle with paprika and garnish with chopped chives if desired.
7. Chill in the refrigerator until ready to serve.

NUTRITIONAL INFORMATION:

Calories: 150 | **Protein:** 12g | **Carbohydrates:** 2g | **Dietary Fiber:** 0g | **Sugars:** 1g | **Fat:** 10g | **Sodium:** 125mg | **Potassium:** 120mg | **Phosphorus:** 180mg

Baked Apple Chips

Yield: 1 serving | **Prep time:** 5 minutes | **Cook time:** 2 hours

INGREDIENTS:

- 1 large apple

DIRECTIONS:

1. Preheat your oven to 200°F (93°C).

2. Core the apple and slice it very thinly, aiming for slices of even thickness to ensure they bake evenly.

3. Arrange the apple slices in a single layer on a baking sheet lined with parchment paper.

4. Bake in the preheated oven for 1 hour, flip the slices, and continue baking for another hour or until the apple slices are dried but still pliable.

5. Remove from the oven and let them cool completely on a wire rack; they will continue to crisp up as they cool.

NUTRITIONAL INFORMATION:

Calories: 95 | **Protein:** 0.5g | **Carbohydrates:** 25g | **Dietary Fiber:** 4.4g | **Sugars:** 19g | **Fat:** 0.3g | **Sodium:** 2mg | **Potassium:** 195mg | **Phosphorus:** 20mg

Chilled Cucumber Soup

Yield: 1 serving | **Prep time:** 10 minutes | **Cook time:** 0 minutes (requires chilling)

INGREDIENTS:

- 1 large cucumber, peeled and roughly chopped
- 1/2 cup plain, non-fat Greek yogurt
- 1/4 cup low-sodium vegetable broth
- 1 tablespoon fresh dill, chopped
- 1 tablespoon lemon juice
- 1 small garlic clove, minced
- Black pepper to taste

DIRECTIONS:

1. Combine the cucumber, Greek yogurt, low-sodium vegetable broth, dill, lemon juice, and garlic in a blender. Blend until smooth.

2. Taste the soup and season with black pepper as needed. For a thinner consistency, you can add a bit of vegetable broth.

3. Chill the soup in the refrigerator for at least 1 hour to allow the flavors to meld and the soup to cool thoroughly.

4. Before serving, give the soup a quick stir. Serve cold, garnished with additional dill if desired.

NUTRITIONAL INFORMATION:

Calories: 120 | **Protein:** 9g | **Carbohydrates:** 16g | **Dietary Fiber:** 2g | **Sugars:** 9g | **Fat:** 3g | **Sodium:** 60mg | **Potassium:** 440mg | **Phosphorus:** 100mg

Fresh Fruit Skewers

Yield: 1 serving | **Prep time:** 10 minutes | **Cook time:** 0 minutes

INGREDIENTS:

- 2 strawberries, halved
- 1/4 cup pineapple chunks
- 1/2 small banana, sliced
- 1/4 cup cantaloupe, cubed
- 2 wooden skewers

DIRECTIONS:

1. Wash the strawberries and peel the banana. Prepare all fruits by cutting them into pieces or chunks that fit easily onto skewers.

2. Thread the fruit onto the skewers, alternating between strawberries, pineapple, banana slices, and cantaloupe cubes to create a colorful variety.

3. Arrange the fruit skewers on a plate. If not serving immediately, cover and refrigerate to keep them fresh.

4. Enjoy as a refreshing, healthy snack or part of a meal.

NUTRITIONAL INFORMATION:

Calories: 150 | **Protein:** 2g | **Carbohydrates:** 38g | **Dietary Fiber:** 4g | **Sugars:** 26g | **Fat:** 0.5g | **Sodium:** 5mg | **Potassium:** 500mg | **Phosphorus:** 30mg

Tuna Salad Stuffed Cherry Tomatoes

Yield: 1 serving | **Prep time:** 15 minutes | **Cook time:** 0 minutes

INGREDIENTS:

- 8 large cherry tomatoes
- 1 (3-ounce) can low-sodium tuna, drained
- 1 tablespoon low-fat mayonnaise
- 1 teaspoon lemon juice
- 1 tablespoon chopped celery
- 1 tablespoon chopped red onion
- Black pepper to taste
- Fresh parsley for garnish (optional)

DIRECTIONS:

1. Slice the tops of the cherry tomatoes and use a small spoon or melon baller to scoop out the insides, creating a hollow space inside each tomato.

2. In a small bowl, mix the drained tuna, low-fat mayonnaise, lemon juice, chopped celery, chopped red onion, and black pepper until well combined.

3. Carefully spoon the tuna mixture into each hollowed-out cherry tomato.

4. Garnish the stuffed tomatoes with fresh parsley if desired.

5. Chill in the refrigerator for about 10 minutes before serving to allow the flavors to meld.

NUTRITIONAL INFORMATION:

Calories: 180 | **Protein:** 22g | **Carbohydrates:** 8g | **Dietary Fiber:** 2g | **Sugars:** 4g | **Fat:** 7g | **Sodium:** 200mg | **Potassium:** 400mg | **Phosphorus:** 250mg

Sliced Radishes with Low-Sodium Soy Sauce Dip

Yield: 1 serving | **Prep time:** 5 minutes | **Cook time:** 0 minutes

INGREDIENTS:

- 1/2 cup radishes, thinly sliced
- 1 tablespoon low-sodium soy sauce
- 1/2 teaspoon sesame oil
- 1/4 teaspoon rice vinegar
- A pinch of black pepper

DIRECTIONS:

1. Wash the radishes under cold water, then slice them thinly.

2. Mix the low-sodium soy sauce, sesame oil, rice vinegar, and black pepper in a small bowl to create the dip.

3. Arrange the sliced radishes on a plate.

4. Serve the radishes with the soy sauce dip on the side for dipping.

NUTRITIONAL INFORMATION:

Calories: 45 | **Protein:** 2g | **Carbohydrates:** 4g | **Dietary Fiber:** 1g | **Sugars:** 2g | **Fat:** 2.5g | **Sodium:** 330mg | **Potassium:** 270mg | **Phosphorus:** 30mg

CHAPTER 9

Desserts

—

Carrot Cake with Cream Cheese Frosting
(Low Sodium)

Yield: 1 serving | **Prep time:** 20 minutes | **Cook time:** 30 minutes

INGREDIENTS:

Cake:
- 1/4 cup all-purpose flour
- 1/4 teaspoon baking powder (low sodium)
- 1/4 teaspoon ground cinnamon
- 1/8 teaspoon ground nutmeg
- 1/8 teaspoon ground ginger
- 1 large egg
- 1/4 cup granulated sugar
- 1/4 cup finely grated carrot
- 1 tablespoon unsweetened applesauce
- 1 tablespoon vegetable oil

Frosting:
- 2 tablespoons cream cheese, softened
- 1 tablespoon unsalted butter, softened
- 1/4 cup powdered sugar
- 1/2 teaspoon vanilla extract

DIRECTIONS:

1. Preheat the oven to 350°F (175°C). Grease and flour a small cake pan or muffin tin.
2. Mix flour, baking powder, cinnamon, nutmeg, and ginger in a bowl.
3. In another bowl, beat the egg with the sugar until light and fluffy. Stir in the grated carrot, applesauce, and vegetable oil.
4. Gradually add the dry ingredients to the wet ingredients, stirring until combined.
5. Pour the batter into the prepared pan and bake for 30 minutes, or until a toothpick inserted into the center comes out clean.
6. For the frosting, beat cream cheese, butter, powdered sugar, and vanilla extract until smooth.
7. Once the cake has cooled, spread the frosting.
8. Serve and enjoy.

NUTRITIONAL INFORMATION:

Calories: 586 | **Protein:** 8.2g | **Carbohydrates:** 83.7g | **Dietary Fiber:** 1.4g | **Sugars:** 64.3g | **Fat:** 26.5g | **Sodium:** 113mg | **Potassium:** 204mg | **Phosphorus:** 135mg

Vanilla Rice Pudding

Yield: 1 serving | **Prep time:** 5 minutes | **Cook time:** 25 minutes

INGREDIENTS:

- 1/4 cup uncooked white rice
- 1 cup water
- 1/2 cup low-fat milk
- 1 tablespoon sugar
- 1/2 teaspoon vanilla extract
- A pinch of salt

DIRECTIONS:

1. In a small saucepan, bring the water to a boil. Add the rice and reduce the heat to low. Cover and simmer for about 20 minutes or until the rice is tender and the water is absorbed.

2. Add the milk, sugar, vanilla extract, and a pinch of salt to the cooked rice. Stir well to combine.

3. Increase the heat to medium-low and cook the mixture, stirring frequently, for about 5 minutes or until the pudding thickens to your desired consistency.

4. Remove from heat and let the rice pudding cool slightly. It can be served warm or chilled, according to your preference.

NUTRITIONAL INFORMATION:

Calories: 220 | **Protein:** 5g | **Carbohydrates:** 45g | **Dietary Fiber:** 0.5g | **Sugars:** 15g | **Fat:** 2g | **Sodium:** 85mg | **Potassium:** 150mg | **Phosphorus:** 100mg

Baked Cinnamon Apples

Yield: 1 serving | **Prep time:** 10 minutes | **Cook time:** 30 minutes

INGREDIENTS:

- 1 medium apple (choose a low-potassium variety like Fuji or Granny Smith)
- 1/2 teaspoon ground cinnamon
- 1 teaspoon unsalted butter (optional)
- 1 teaspoon honey (optional, use in moderation)

DIRECTIONS:

1. Preheat your oven to 350°F (175°C).

2. Wash the apple and remove the core and seeds. Leave the skin intact.

3. Slice the apple into thin rings or wedges.

4. In a bowl, toss the apple slices with ground cinnamon until they are evenly coated.

5. If desired, lightly grease a small baking dish with unsalted butter to prevent sticking. Place the cinnamon-coated apple slices in the baking dish.

6. Drizzle honey sparingly over the apples for added sweetness (optional).

7. Cover the baking dish with aluminum foil.

8. Bake in the oven for about 30 minutes or until the apples are tender but not mushy. Check with a fork for desired tenderness.

9. Remove from the oven and let it cool slightly before serving.

NUTRITIONAL INFORMATION:

Calories: 100 | **Protein:** 0.5g | **Carbohydrates:** 26g | **Dietary Fiber:** 4g | **Sugars:** 19g | **Fat:** 0.5g | **Sodium:** 0mg | **Potassium:** 150mg | **Phosphorus:** 10mg

Honey-Glazed Grilled Peaches

Yield: 1 serving | **Prep time:** 5 minutes | **Cook time:** 10 minutes

INGREDIENTS:

- 1 giant peach, halved and pitted
- 1 tablespoon honey
- 1/2 teaspoon cinnamon
- 1 teaspoon olive oil (for grill pan)

DIRECTIONS:

1. Preheat your grill pan over medium heat and brush it with olive oil to prevent the peaches from sticking.

2. In a small bowl, mix the honey and cinnamon. Brush the mixture over the cut sides of the peach halves.

3. Place the peach halves, cut side down, on the grill pan. Grill for 4-5 minutes or until the peaches have grill marks.

4. Flip the peaches over and grill for another 4-5 minutes or until tender and heated.

5. Serve warm, optionally, with a dollop of Greek yogurt or a sprinkle of chopped nuts for added texture and flavor.

NUTRITIONAL INFORMATION:

Calories: 175 | **Protein:** 1.7g | **Carbohydrates:** 35.3g | **Dietary Fiber:** 3.3g | **Sugars:** 32.5g | **Fat:** 4.9g | **Sodium:** 1mg | **Potassium:** 355mg | **Phosphorus:** 32mg

Blueberry Crisp with Oat Topping

Yield: 1 serving | **Prep time:** 10 minutes | **Cook time:** 25 minutes

INGREDIENTS:

- 1/2 cup fresh blueberries
- 1 tablespoon granulated sugar
- 1/4 teaspoon vanilla extract
- 2 tablespoons rolled oats
- 1 tablespoon all-purpose flour
- 1 tablespoon brown sugar
- 1/4 teaspoon ground cinnamon
- 1 tablespoon unsalted butter, chilled and cubed

DIRECTIONS:

1. Preheat the oven to 375°F (190°C). Lightly grease a small baking dish.

2. Mix the blueberries with granulated sugar and vanilla extract. Pour the mixture into the prepared baking dish.

3. Combine rolled oats, all-purpose flour, brown sugar, and ground cinnamon in another bowl. Add the cubed butter and use your fingers to mix until the mixture resembles coarse crumbs.

4. Sprinkle the oat mixture over the blueberries in the dish.

5. Bake in the oven for 25 minutes or until the topping is golden brown and the blueberries are bubbly.

6. Let cool slightly before serving.

NUTRITIONAL INFORMATION:

Calories: 286 | **Protein:** 2.4g | **Carbohydrates:** 46.9g | **Dietary Fiber:** 3.4g | **Sugars:** 34.5g | **Fat:** 11.2g | **Sodium:** 6mg | **Potassium:** 85mg | **Phosphorus:** 45mg

Lemon Sorbet

Yield: 1 serving | **Prep time:** 10 minutes | **Cook time:** 0 minutes (plus freezing time)

INGREDIENTS:

- 1/2 cup water
- 1/4 cup sugar
- 1/2 cup fresh lemon juice (about 2-3 lemons)
- 1 teaspoon lemon zest

DIRECTIONS:

1. In a small saucepan, combine water and sugar. Heat over medium heat, stirring until the sugar has completely dissolved. Remove from heat and let it cool to room temperature.
2. Stir in the lemon juice and zest once the syrup cools.
3. Pour the mixture into a shallow dish and freeze until firm, stirring every 30 minutes to break up ice crystals, for about 2-3 hours.
4. Once frozen, use a fork to scrape the sorbet into fluffy crystals.
5. Serve immediately in a chilled bowl or store in the freezer until ready to serve.

NUTRITIONAL INFORMATION:

Calories: 194 | **Protein:** 0.3g | **Carbohydrates:** 50.3g | **Dietary Fiber:** 0.2g | **Sugars:** 49.4g | **Fat:** 0.1g | **Sodium:** 3mg | **Potassium:** 75mg | **Phosphorus:** 2mg

Almond Flour Shortbread Cookies

Yield: 1 serving | **Prep time:** 10 minutes | **Cook time:** 12 minutes

INGREDIENTS:

- 1/4 cup almond flour
- 1 tablespoon unsalted butter, softened
- 1 tablespoon powdered sugar
- 1/4 teaspoon vanilla extract

DIRECTIONS:

1. Preheat your oven to 350°F (175°C) and line a baking sheet with parchment paper.
2. Combine almond flour, softened butter, powdered sugar, and vanilla extract in a mixing bowl. Stir until a soft dough forms.
3. Shape the dough into a ball, then flatten it into a disk on the parchment paper. Cut into desired shapes using a knife or cookie cutter.
4. Bake in the oven for 12 minutes or until the edges are slightly golden brown.
5. Let the cookies cool on the baking sheet for a few minutes before transferring them to a wire rack to cool completely.

NUTRITIONAL INFORMATION:

Calories: 234 | **Protein:** 5g | **Carbohydrates:** 11g | **Dietary Fiber:** 2g | **Sugars:** 7g | **Fat:** 20g | **Sodium:** 2mg | **Potassium:** 5mg | **Phosphorus:** 98mg

Watermelon and Feta Salad

Yield: 1 serving | **Prep time:** 10 minutes | **Cook time:** 0 minutes

INGREDIENTS:

- 1 cup cubed watermelon
- 1/4 cup crumbled feta cheese
- 1 tablespoon chopped fresh mint leaves
- 1 teaspoon olive oil
- 1 teaspoon balsamic vinegar
- A pinch of black pepper

DIRECTIONS:

1. Combine the cubed watermelon and crumbled feta cheese in a serving bowl.
2. Sprinkle the chopped fresh mint leaves over the watermelon and feta mixture.
3. Drizzle with olive oil and balsamic vinegar.
4. Season with a pinch of black pepper to taste.
5. Gently toss all the ingredients together until the salad is well-mixed.
6. Serve immediately or chill in the refrigerator for a refreshing and cool treat.

NUTRITIONAL INFORMATION:

Calories: 156 | **Protein:** 4.5g | **Carbohydrates:** 14g | **Dietary Fiber:** 0.6g | **Sugars:** 12g | **Fat:** 9.5g | **Sodium:** 256mg | **Potassium:** 170mg | **Phosphorus:** 100mg

Lemon Ricotta Cheesecake
(Low-Phosphorus)

Yield: 1 serving | **Prep time:** 20 minutes | **Cook time:** 45 minutes

INGREDIENTS:

- 1/2 cup low-fat ricotta cheese
- 2 tablespoons granulated sugar
- 1 large egg
- 1/2 teaspoon vanilla extract
- 1 teaspoon lemon zest
- 1 tablespoon lemon juice
- 1 tablespoon all-purpose flour

DIRECTIONS:

1. Preheat the oven to 350°F (175°C). Lightly grease a small baking dish or springform pan.
2. Mix the ricotta cheese and sugar in a mixing bowl until smooth.
3. Beat in the egg, then mix in the vanilla extract, lemon zest, and lemon juice until well combined.
4. Fold in the flour, making sure not to overmix.
5. Pour the mixture into the prepared baking dish or pan.
6. Bake in the oven for 45 minutes or until the center is set and the top is lightly golden.
7. Let the cheesecake cool in the pan on a wire rack, then refrigerate until chilled, at least 4 hours or overnight.
8. Serve chilled, optionally garnished with extra lemon zest or fresh berries.

NUTRITIONAL INFORMATION:

Calories: 245 | **Protein:** 14g | **Carbohydrates:** 26g | **Dietary Fiber:** 0.2g | **Sugars:** 25g | **Fat:** 10g | **Sodium:** 150mg | **Potassium:** 155mg | **Phosphorus:** 190mg

Baked Pears with Honey and Cinnamon

Yield: 1 serving | **Prep time:** 5 minutes | **Cook time:** 25 minutes

INGREDIENTS:

- 1 large pear, halved and cored
- 1 tablespoon honey
- 1/2 teaspoon ground cinnamon
- A pinch of ground nutmeg (optional)
- 1/4 cup water

DIRECTIONS:

1. Preheat your oven to 350°F (175°C).
2. Place the pear halves with the cut side up in a baking dish. Drizzle with honey and sprinkle with cinnamon and nutmeg, if using.
3. Add water to the bottom of the dish to prevent the pears from sticking and to add moisture while they bake.
4. Bake in the preheated oven for 25 minutes or until the pears are tender and cooked.
5. Serve warm; spoon any of the baking dish's juices over the pears.

NUTRITIONAL INFORMATION:

Calories: 162 | **Protein:** 0.6g | **Carbohydrates:** 43.2g | **Dietary Fiber:** 5.5g | **Sugars:** 32.7g | **Fat:** 0.3g | **Sodium:** 2mg | **Potassium:** 206mg | **Phosphorus:** 20mg

Poached Pears in White Wine

Yield: 1 serving | **Prep time:** 10 minutes | **Cook time:** 25 minutes

INGREDIENTS:

- 1 large pear, peeled, halved, and cored
- 1/2 cup white wine
- 1/4 cup water
- 2 tablespoons sugar
- 1 cinnamon stick
- 1 strip of lemon zest

DIRECTIONS:

1. Combine the white wine, water, sugar, cinnamon stick, and lemon zest in a small saucepan. Bring to a simmer over medium heat.
2. Add the pear halves to the saucepan, ensuring the liquid covers them. If not, add a little more water until they are just covered.
3. Simmer gently for 25 minutes or until the pears are tender, turning occasionally to ensure even cooking.
4. Carefully remove the pears from the liquid and place them on a serving plate.
5. Increase the heat under the saucepan and reduce the cooking liquid by half, about 10 minutes, to create a syrup.
6. Pour the reduced syrup over the pears before serving.
7. Serve warm or allow to cool to room temperature.

NUTRITIONAL INFORMATION:

Calories: 236 | **Protein:** 0.5g | **Carbohydrates:** 38g | **Dietary Fiber:** 4g | **Sugars:** 29g | **Fat:** 0.2g | **Sodium:** 5mg | **Potassium:** 206mg | **Phosphorus:** 20mg

Mixed Berry Salad with Mint

Yield: 1 serving | **Prep time:** 10 minutes | **Cook time:** 0 minutes

INGREDIENTS:

- 1/2 cup fresh strawberries, hulled and halved
- 1/2 cup fresh blueberries
- 1/2 cup fresh raspberries
- 1/2 cup fresh blackberries
- 1 tablespoon fresh mint leaves, finely chopped
- 1 tablespoon honey (optional)
- 1 teaspoon fresh lemon juice (optional)

DIRECTIONS:

1. In a large mixing bowl, gently combine the strawberries, blueberries, raspberries, and blackberries.
2. In a small bowl, mix the chopped mint leaves with honey and lemon juice, if using, until well combined.
3. Drizzle the mint mixture over the berries and gently toss to coat.
4. Let the salad sit for about 5 minutes to allow the flavors to meld.
5. Serve the salad in a bowl, garnished with additional mint leaves if desired

NUTRITIONAL INFORMATION:

Calories: 122 | **Protein:** 2g | **Carbohydrates:** 31g | **Dietary Fiber:** 8g | **Sugars:** 20g | **Fat:** 0.7g | **Sodium:** 3mg | **Potassium:** 233mg | **Phosphorus:** 35mg

Apple Crumble with Oat Topping

Yield: 1 serving | **Prep time:** 15 minutes | **Cook time:** 30 minutes

INGREDIENTS:

- 1 large apple, peeled, cored, and sliced
- 1 tablespoon granulated sugar
- 1/2 teaspoon ground cinnamon
- 2 tablespoons rolled oats
- 1 tablespoon all-purpose flour
- 1 tablespoon brown sugar
- 1 tablespoon unsalted butter, cold and cubed

DIRECTIONS:

1. Preheat the oven to 350°F (175°C). Lightly grease a small baking dish.
2. toss the sliced apple with granulated sugar and cinnamon in a mixing bowl. Place the apple mixture in the prepared baking dish.
3. Mix rolled oats, all-purpose flour, and brown sugar in another bowl. Add the cubed butter and use your fingers to rub the butter into the oat mixture until it resembles coarse crumbs.
4. Sprinkle the oat mixture evenly over the apples in the baking dish.
5. Bake in the oven for about 30 minutes or until the topping is golden brown and the apples are tender.
6. Allow to cool slightly before serving.

NUTRITIONAL INFORMATION:

Calories: 324 | **Protein:** 2.5g | **Carbohydrates:** 58.5g | **Dietary Fiber:** 4.7g | **Sugars:** 42.8g | **Fat:** 11.7g | **Sodium:** 2mg | **Potassium:** 195mg | **Phosphorus:** 40mg

Pineapple Sorbet

Yield: 1 serving | **Prep time:** 10 minutes | **Cook time:** 0 minutes (requires freezing time)

INGREDIENTS:

- 1 cup frozen pineapple chunks
- 2 tablespoons sugar
- 1/4 cup water
- 1 teaspoon lime juice

DIRECTIONS:

1. Combine the frozen pineapple chunks, sugar, water, and lime juice in a blender. Blend until smooth.
2. Taste and adjust sweetness if necessary, blending again if more sugar is added.
3. Transfer the mixture to a freezer-safe container and freeze until firm, about 2-3 hours, stirring occasionally to break up ice crystals.
4. Once frozen to the desired consistency, serve with a spoon or ice cream scoop.
5. Enjoy immediately as a refreshing frozen dessert.

NUTRITIONAL INFORMATION:

Calories: 132 | **Protein:** 0.5g | **Carbohydrates:** 34.2g | **Dietary Fiber:** 2g | **Sugars:** 31.2g | **Fat:** 0.2g | **Sodium:** 3mg | **Potassium:** 120mg | **Phosphorus:** 2mg

Low-Phosphorus Chocolate Mousse

Yield: 1 serving | **Prep time:** 15 minutes | **Cook time:** 0 minutes
(requires chilling for at least 2 hours)

INGREDIENTS:

- 1/4 cup heavy whipping cream
- 1 tablespoon unsweetened cocoa powder
- 1 tablespoon sugar
- 1/4 teaspoon vanilla extract

DIRECTIONS:

1. In a chilled mixing bowl, add the heavy whipping cream and whip until soft peaks form.
2. Sift the cocoa powder and sugar, then add the vanilla extract. Continue to whip until the mixture is well combined and forms stiff peaks.
3. Spoon the chocolate mousse into a serving dish or glass.
4. Chill in the refrigerator for at least 2 hours or until set.
5. Serve chilled, optionally garnished with a sprinkle of cocoa powder or a few fresh berries for added flavor.

NUTRITIONAL INFORMATION:

Calories: 245 | **Protein:** 14g | **Carbohydrates:** 26g | **Dietary Fiber:** 0.2g | **Sugars:** 25g | **Fat:** 10g | **Sodium:** 150mg | **Potassium:** 155mg | **Phosphorus:** 190mg

Coconut Rice Pudding

Yield: 1 serving | **Prep time:** 5 minutes | **Cook time:** 25 minutes

INGREDIENTS:

- 1/4 cup uncooked white rice
- 1 cup coconut milk (use light coconut milk for lower fat content)
- 1 tablespoon sugar
- 1/4 teaspoon vanilla extract
- A pinch of salt
- Ground cinnamon for garnish (optional)

DIRECTIONS:

1. Rinse the rice under cold water until the water runs clear.
2. Combine the rinsed rice, coconut milk, and a pinch of salt in a small saucepan. Bring the mixture to a boil over medium heat.
3. Once boiling, reduce the heat to low and cover the pan. Simmer for about 20 minutes or until the rice is tender and the mixture has thickened.
4. Remove from heat and stir in the sugar and vanilla extract.
5. Transfer the rice pudding to a serving dish and cool slightly. It can be served warm or chilled.
6. Garnish with a sprinkle of ground cinnamon before serving, if desired.

NUTRITIONAL INFORMATION:

Calories: 385 | **Protein:** 5g | **Carbohydrates:** 44g | **Dietary Fiber:** 0.5g | **Sugars:** 9g | **Fat:** 21g | **Sodium:** 15mg | **Potassium:** 260mg | **Phosphorus:** 100mg

Low-Potassium Berry Parfait

Yield: 1 serving | **Prep time:** 10 minutes | **Cook time:** 0 minutes

INGREDIENTS:

- 1/2 cup low-potassium berries (such as blueberries, strawberries, or raspberries)
- 1/2 cup low-potassium yogurt (choose a renal-friendly brand)
- 2 tablespoons granola (low-potassium or homemade)
- 1 teaspoon honey (optional, use in moderation)

DIRECTIONS:

1. Wash and prepare the berries. If using strawberries, remove the stems and slice them into smaller pieces.
2. lay half of the low-potassium yogurt in a serving glass or bowl.
3. Add a layer of half of the prepared berries on top of the yogurt.
4. Sprinkle one tablespoon of granola over the berries.
5. Repeat the layers with the remaining yogurt, berries, and another tablespoon of granola.
6. If desired, drizzle honey sparingly over the top for a touch of sweetness (optional).
7. Serve immediately or refrigerate until ready to enjoy.

NUTRITIONAL INFORMATION:

Calories: 200 | **Protein:** 6g | **Carbohydrates:** 38g | **Dietary Fiber:** 5g | **Sugars:** 17g | **Fat:** 3g | **Sodium:** 50mg | **Potassium:** 150mg | **Phosphorus:** 80mg

Grilled Banana with Honey Glaze

Yield: 1 serving | **Prep time:** 5 minutes | **Cook time:** 10 minutes

INGREDIENTS:

- 1 banana, peeled
- 1 tablespoon honey
- A pinch of ground cinnamon
- A small pinch of salt (optional)

DIRECTIONS:

1. Preheat the grill to medium-high heat.
2. Slice the banana in half lengthwise.
3. In a small bowl, mix the honey with the cinnamon and salt, if using.
4. Brush the honey mixture over the cut sides of the banana halves.
5. Place the banana halves, cut side down, on the grill. Grill for about 5 minutes or until grill marks appear.
6. Carefully turn the bananas over and grill for another 4-5 minutes or until the bananas are soft and warm throughout.
7. Serve immediately, with an extra drizzle of honey if desired.

NUTRITIONAL INFORMATION:

Calories: 151 | **Protein:** 1.3g | **Carbohydrates:** 39.3g | **Dietary Fiber:** 3.1g | **Sugars:** 27.2g | **Fat:** 0.4g | **Sodium:** 1mg | **Potassium:** 422mg | **Phosphorus:** 26mg

Peach Cobbler with Low-Phosphorus Biscuit Topping

Yield: 1 serving | **Prep time:** 15 minutes | **Cook time:** 25 minutes

INGREDIENTS:

- Peach Filling:
- 1 giant peach, peeled and sliced
- 1 tablespoon granulated sugar
- 1/4 teaspoon ground cinnamon
- 1 teaspoon cornstarch
- Biscuit Topping:
- 1/4 cup all-purpose flour
- 1/2 teaspoon baking powder (low-phosphorus)
- 1 tablespoon unsalted butter, cold
- 2 tablespoons milk
- 1 tablespoon granulated sugar

DIRECTIONS:

1. Preheat the oven to 375°F (190°C). Grease a small baking dish.
2. In a bowl, combine the peach slices, one tablespoon of sugar, cinnamon, and cornstarch. Toss until the peaches are evenly coated. Transfer the mixture to the prepared baking dish.
3. In another bowl, mix the flour and baking powder. Cut in the cold butter until the mixture resembles coarse crumbs. Stir in the milk and one tablespoon of sugar to form a soft dough.
4. Drop spoonfuls of the biscuit dough over the peach mixture in the baking dish.
5. Bake in the oven for 25 minutes or until the biscuit topping is golden and the peach filling is bubbly.
6. Let cool slightly before serving.

NUTRITIONAL INFORMATION:

Calories: 340 | **Protein:** 4g | **Carbohydrates:** 58g | **Dietary Fiber:** 3g | **Sugars:** 34g | **Fat:** 12g | **Sodium:** 95mg | **Potassium:** 250mg | **Phosphorus:** 100mg

Angel Food Cake with Fresh Strawberries

Yield: 1 serving | **Prep time:** 15 minutes | **Cook time:** 0 minutes

INGREDIENTS:

- 1 slice of store-bought angel food cake (approximately 28g)
- 1/2 cup fresh strawberries, sliced
- 1 tablespoon powdered sugar (optional for dusting)

DIRECTIONS:

1. Rinse the fresh strawberries under cold water and slice them thinly.
2. Place the slice of angel food cake on a serving plate.
3. Arrange the sliced strawberries on top of the angel food cake.
4. dust the top with powdered sugar for a sweet finish.
5. Serve immediately and enjoy this light and refreshing dessert.

NUTRITIONAL INFORMATION:

Calories: 99 | **Protein:** 2.2g | **Carbohydrates:** 22.8g | **Dietary Fiber:** 1.7g | **Sugars:** 13.9g | **Fat:** 0.3g | **Sodium:** 211mg | **Potassium:** 187mg | **Phosphorus:** 23mg

Baked Custard

(Low Phosphorus)

Yield: 1 serving | **Prep time:** 10 minutes | **Cook time:** 45 minutes

INGREDIENTS:

- 1 large egg
- 2 tablespoons granulated sugar
- 1/2 cup milk (use low-phosphorus milk substitute if necessary)
- 1/2 teaspoon vanilla extract
- A pinch of ground nutmeg

DIRECTIONS:

1. Preheat the oven to 325°F (165°C). Have a small baking dish ready and a larger baking pan for a water bath.
2. In a bowl, whisk together the egg and sugar until well combined.
3. Heat the milk until it's warm but not boiling, then gradually add it to the egg mixture, stirring constantly. Stir in the vanilla extract.
4. Pour the mixture into the small baking dish. Sprinkle the top with a pinch of ground nutmeg.
5. Place the small dish in the larger baking pan. Pour hot water into the larger pan until it comes halfway up the sides of the small dish.
6. Bake in the oven for 45 minutes or until the custard is set but still jiggly in the center.
7. Carefully remove it from the oven and the water bath, then let it cool to room temperature. Chill in the refrigerator before serving.

NUTRITIONAL INFORMATION:

Calories: 202 | **Protein:** 6.7g | **Carbohydrates:** 29.3g | **Dietary Fiber:** 0g | **Sugars:** 29g | **Fat:** 7.3g | **Sodium:** 106mg | **Potassium:** 192mg | **Phosphorus:** 129mg

Strawberry Gelatin with Whipped Topping

Yield: 1 serving | **Prep time:** 10 minutes | **Cook time:** 0 minutes (plus chilling time)

INGREDIENTS:

- 1/2 cup boiling water
- 1/2 packet sugar-free strawberry gelatin (about 2g)
- 1/2 cup cold water
- 1/4 cup whipped topping

DIRECTIONS:

1. In a bowl, stir the sugar-free strawberry gelatin in the boiling water until completely dissolved.
2. Add the cold water to the gelatin mixture and stir well.
3. Pour the gelatin mixture into a serving dish or mold. Refrigerate until set, about 2-3 hours.
4. Once set, top the strawberry gelatin with whipped topping before serving.
5. Serve chilled as a refreshing dessert.

NUTRITIONAL INFORMATION:

Calories: 60 | **Protein:** 1g | **Carbohydrates:** 8g | **Dietary Fiber:** 0g | **Sugars:** 1g | **Fat:** 3g | **Sodium:** 55mg | **Potassium:** 10mg | **Phosphorus:** 0mg

Low-Sodium Apple Pie

Yield: 1 serving | **Prep time:** 30 minutes | **Cook time:** 45 minutes

INGREDIENTS:

- 1 medium apple, peeled and sliced
- 1/2 tablespoon all-purpose flour
- 2 tablespoons granulated sugar
- 1/4 teaspoon ground cinnamon
- 1/8 teaspoon ground nutmeg
- 1 low-sodium pie crust (store-bought or homemade without salt)
- 1 teaspoon unsalted butter, cut into small pieces
- 1 tablespoon milk (for brushing the crust)

DIRECTIONS:

1. Preheat the oven to 375°F (190°C).
2. Combine the sliced apples, flour, sugar, cinnamon, and nutmeg in a bowl. Toss until the apples are evenly coated.
3. Place the apple mixture into the pie crust, spreading evenly. Dot the top with pieces of unsalted butter.
4. Cover the filling with another pie crust or create a lattice top. Seal the edges by crimping with a fork or your fingers.
5. Brush the top crust lightly with milk to help it brown.
6. Make a few slits in the top crust to allow steam to escape.
7. Bake in the oven for 45 minutes or until the crust is golden brown and the filling is bubbly.
8. Let the pie cool for at least 2 hours before serving to allow the filling to set.

NUTRITIONAL INFORMATION:

Calories: 350 | **Protein:** 3g | **Carbohydrates:** 58g | **Dietary Fiber:** 3g | **Sugars:** 28g | **Fat:** 12g | **Sodium:** 30mg | **Potassium:** 150mg | **Phosphorus:** 40mg

Berry and Yogurt Smoothie

Yield: 1 serving | **Prep time:** 5 minutes | **Cook time:** 0 minutes

INGREDIENTS:

- 1/2 cup fresh strawberries
- 1/2 cup fresh blueberries
- 1/2 banana
- 1/2 cup plain, low-fat yogurt
- 1/4 cup water or as needed for blending
- 1 teaspoon honey (optional)

DIRECTIONS:

1. Wash the strawberries and blueberries thoroughly under cold water.
2. Peel the banana and cut it into slices.
3. Combine the strawberries, blueberries, banana slices, and yogurt in a blender.
4. Add water to help with the blending process. Blend on high until smooth.
5. Taste the smoothie and add honey if a sweeter taste is desired. Blend again for a few seconds to incorporate the honey.
6. Pour the smoothie into a glass and serve immediately.

NUTRITIONAL INFORMATION:

Calories: 192 | **Protein:** 6g | **Carbohydrates:** 40g | **Dietary Fiber:** 5g | **Sugars:** 28g | **Fat:** 2g | **Sodium:** 70mg | **Potassium:** 532mg | **Phosphorus:** 159mg

Chia Seed Pudding with Almond Milk

Yield: 1 serving | **Prep time:** 5 minutes | **Cook time:** 0 minutes
(requires at least 4 hours of refrigeration)

INGREDIENTS:

- 3 tablespoons chia seeds
- 3/4 cup unsweetened almond milk
- 1/2 teaspoon vanilla extract
- 1 tablespoon maple syrup or honey (optional for sweetness)
- Fresh fruit for topping (optional)

DIRECTIONS:

1. Combine the chia seeds, almond milk, vanilla extract, and maple syrup or honey in a small bowl or jar. Stir well to mix.
2. Cover and refrigerate for at least 4 hours, or overnight, until the mixture thickens and becomes pudding-like.
3. Stir the pudding again before serving. Add more almond milk to reach your desired consistency if the pudding is too thick.
4. Top with fresh fruit of your choice, such as berries or sliced banana, just before serving.
5. Enjoy this healthy and nourishing breakfast or dessert.

NUTRITIONAL INFORMATION:

Calories: 210 | **Protein:** 6g | **Carbohydrates:** 24g | **Dietary Fiber:** 10g | **Sugars:** 8g (varies if additional sweeteners or fruits are added) | **Fat:** 12g | **Sodium:** 95mg | **Potassium:** 150mg | **Phosphorus:** 240mg

CHAPTER 10

Beverages

———

Blueberry Smoothie
(Low Potassium)

Yield: 1 serving | **Prep time:** 5 minutes | **Cook time:** 0 minutes

INGREDIENTS:

- 1/2 cup fresh or frozen blueberries
- 1/2 cup low-fat milk (or a low-potassium milk substitute, such as rice milk)
- 1/4 cup plain, low-fat yogurt
- 1 tablespoon honey (optional, depending on sweetness preference)
- A few ice cubes (if using fresh blueberries)

DIRECTIONS:

1. Place the blueberries, milk, yogurt, and honey (if using) into a blender.
2. Add ice cubes if you use fresh blueberries to make the smoothie cold.
3. Blend on high until smooth and creamy.
4. Taste the smoothie and add more honey if a sweeter smoothie is desired.
5. Pour the smoothie into a glass and serve immediately.

NUTRITIONAL INFORMATION:

Calories: 155 | **Protein:** 5g | **Carbohydrates:** 28g | **Dietary Fiber:** 2g | **Sugars:** 25g (varies with honey addition) | **Fat:** 2g | **Sodium:** 60mg | **Potassium:** 233mg | **Phosphorus:** 125mg

Homemade Almond Milk
(Unsweetened)

Yield: 1 serving | **Prep time:** 10 minutes | **Cook time:** 0 minutes (plus soaking time)

INGREDIENTS:

- 1/4 cup raw almonds
- 1 cup water (for soaking) + 1 cup water (for blending)

DIRECTIONS:

1. Place the almonds in a bowl and cover with 1 cup of water. Let them soak overnight, or for at least 12 hours, to soften.
2. Drain and rinse the almonds after soaking. Discard the soaking water.
3. Place the soaked almonds and 1 cup of fresh water in a blender.
4. Blend on high speed for 2 minutes or until the mixture is smooth and creamy.
5. Place a nut milk bag or a fine mesh sieve lined with cheesecloth over a bowl and pour the almond mixture through it to strain out the almond pulp.
6. Squeeze or press the nut milk bag or cheesecloth to extract as much liquid as possible.
7. Transfer the homemade almond milk to a clean bottle or jar and refrigerate. Use within 2-3 days for best freshness.
8. Optional: For flavored almond milk, you can add vanilla extract, cinnamon, or sweeteners to taste before blending.

NUTRITIONAL INFORMATION:

Calories: 60 | **Protein:** 2g | **Carbohydrates:** 2g | **Dietary Fiber:** 1g | **Sugars:** 0g | **Fat:** 5g | **Sodium:** 8mg | **Potassium:** 75mg | **Phosphorus:** 90mg

Lemon-Lime Infused Water

Yield: 1 serving | **Prep time:** 5 minutes | **Cook time:** 0 minutes

INGREDIENTS:

- 1 cup of water
- 2 slices of lemon
- 2 slices of lime

DIRECTIONS:

1. Fill a glass or jar with 1 cup of water.
2. Add the slices of lemon and lime to the water.
3. Let the water sit in the refrigerator for at least an hour to allow the flavors to infuse. For a more spicy taste, you can leave it overnight.
4. Once infused to your liking, remove the slices of lemon and lime. You can add fresh slices for garnish if desired.
5. Serve the lemon-lime-infused water chilled for a refreshing drink.

NUTRITIONAL INFORMATION:

Calories: 10 | **Protein:** 0g | **Carbohydrates:** 3g | **Dietary Fiber:** 0.5g | **Sugars:** 1g | **Fat:** 0g | **Sodium:** 2mg | **Potassium:** 35mg | **Phosphorus:** 0mg

Apple Cider
(Unsweetened)

Yield: 1 serving | **Prep time:** 15 minutes | **Cook time:** 2 hours

INGREDIENTS:

- 4 large apples, assorted types, quartered
- 4 cups water
- 2 tablespoons lemon juice
- Optional spices: 1 cinnamon stick, two cloves

DIRECTIONS:

1. Combine the quartered apples, water, lemon juice, and optional spices in a large pot. Bring the mixture to a boil.

2. Once boiling, reduce the heat to low and cover the pot. Let it simmer for 2 hours to let the apples soften, and the flavors meld.

3. After simmering, use a potato masher or spoon to mash the cooked apples to release more flavor.

4. Place a fine mesh strainer with cheesecloth over a large bowl. Pour the apple mixture through the sieve to separate the liquid from the apple solids. Press or squeeze the solids to extract as much liquid as possible.

5. Discard the solids. If desired, strain the cider again for a more precise liquid.

6. Allow the cider to cool to room temperature, then refrigerate until cold.

7. Serve the apple cider chilled. Optional: garnish with a cinnamon stick or an apple slice.

NUTRITIONAL INFORMATION:

Calories: 95 | **Protein:** 0.5g | **Carbohydrates:** 25g | **Dietary Fiber:** 4g | **Sugars:** 18g (naturally occurring) | **Fat:** 0.3g | **Sodium:** 5mg | **Potassium:** 195mg | **Phosphorus:** 20mg

Pear Nectar
(Diluted)

Yield: 1 serving | **Prep time:** 5 minutes | **Cook time:** 0 minutes

INGREDIENTS:

- 1/2 cup pear nectar (unsweetened)
- 1/2 cup water

DIRECTIONS:

1. In a glass, combine the pear nectar and water.

2. Stir the mixture well to ensure it's thoroughly combined.

3. Add ice cubes if desired for a chilled beverage.

4. Optionally, add a slice of lemon or lime for a hint of citrus flavor.

5. Serve immediately for a refreshing drink.

NUTRITIONAL INFORMATION:

Calories: 60 | **Protein:** 0g | **Carbohydrates:** 15g | **Dietary Fiber:** 0g | **Sugars:** 14g | **Fat:** 0g | **Sodium:** 10mg | **Potassium:** 120mg | **Phosphorus:** 15mg

Peach Iced Tea
(Unsweetened)

Yield: 1 serving | **Prep time:** 10 minutes | **Cook time:** 5 minutes
(plus cooling and chilling time)

INGREDIENTS:

- 1 cup water
- 1 black tea bag (or green tea for a lighter option)
- 1/2 fresh peach, sliced
- Ice cubes

DIRECTIONS:

1. Bring 1 cup of water to a boil in a small saucepan or kettle.
2. Place the tea bag in a large cup or mug. Pour the boiling water over the tea bag and let it steep for 3-5 minutes, depending on how strong you prefer your tea.
3. While the tea steeps, muddle the peach slices in a separate cup to release their juice and flavor.
4. Remove the tea bag from the water after steeping and let the tea cool to room temperature.
5. Once the tea has cooled, strain the muddled peach slices into the tea, pressing to extract as much peach flavor as possible.
6. Fill a tall glass with ice cubes and pour the peach-infused tea over the ice.
7. Stir well and enjoy the refreshing taste of unsweetened peach iced tea.

NUTRITIONAL INFORMATION:

Calories: 30 | **Protein:** 0.5g | **Carbohydrates:** 7.5g | **Dietary Fiber:** 1g | **Sugars:** 6.5g (naturally occurring from the peach) | **Fat:** 0g | **Sodium:** 2mg | **Potassium:** 90mg | **Phosphorus:** 10mg

Raspberry Lemonade
(Sugar-Free)

Yield: 1 serving | **Prep time:** 10 minutes | **Cook time:** 0 minutes

INGREDIENTS:

- 1/2 cup fresh raspberries
- Juice of 1 large lemon (about 1/4 cup)
- 1 cup cold water
- Sweetener to taste (use a kidney-friendly, sugar-free option such as stevia or erythritol)
- Ice cubes (optional)

DIRECTIONS:

1. Combine the fresh raspberries, lemon juice, and a suitable amount of sugar-free sweetener in a blender. Blend until smooth.
2. Strain the raspberry-lemon mixture through a fine mesh sieve into a glass to remove the seeds. Press on the solids to extract as much liquid as possible.
3. Add cold water to the strained juice and stir well to combine. Adjust the sweetness if necessary by adding more sweetener.
4. Add ice cubes to the glass if desired and serve immediately.
5. Optional: Garnish with a few whole raspberries or a slice of lemon on the rim of the glass for a decorative touch.

NUTRITIONAL INFORMATION:

Calories: 32 | **Protein:** 1g | **Carbohydrates:** 8g | **Dietary Fiber:** 4g | **Sugars:** 1g (naturally occurring in raspberries, varies with the type of sweetener used) | **Fat:** 0.5g | **Sodium:** 1mg | **Potassium:** 115mg | **Phosphorus:** 20mg

Carrot-Ginger Juice
(Homemade)

Yield: 1 serving | **Prep time:** 10 minutes | **Cook time:** 0 minutes

INGREDIENTS:

- 2 large carrots, peeled
- 1/2 inch piece of ginger, peeled
- 1/2 cup water

DIRECTIONS:

1. Wash and peel the carrots and ginger. Chop them into smaller pieces to fit into your juicer.
2. Place the chopped carrots and ginger into the juicer.
3. Add water to the juicer to help extract the juice more efficiently if your juicer requires it.
4. Turn on the juicer and push the carrots and ginger through, collecting the juice in a container.
5. Once all the juice is extracted, stir the juice to ensure the flavors are well combined.
6. Serve the juice immediately for the best flavor and nutritional benefits.
7. Optional: For a smoother juice, strain it through a fine mesh sieve to remove any pulp.

NUTRITIONAL INFORMATION:

Calories: 70 | **Protein:** 1.5g | **Carbohydrates:** 16g | **Dietary Fiber:** 4.5g | **Sugars:** 9g | **Fat:** 0.2g | **Sodium:** 86mg | **Potassium:** 410mg | **Phosphorus:** 45mg

Herbal Tea
(Unsweetened)

Yield: 1 serving | **Prep time:** 5 minutes | **Cook time:** 5 minutes

INGREDIENTS:

- 1 cup water
- 1 herbal tea bag (e.g., chamomile, peppermint, or hibiscus)

DIRECTIONS:

1. Boil 1 cup of water in a kettle or pot.
2. Place the herbal tea bag in a mug.
3. Once the water reaches a rolling boil, pour it over the tea bag in the mug.
4. Let the tea steep for 3-5 minutes, depending on how strong you like your tea.
5. Remove the tea bag from the mug. If you prefer a milder flavor, steep for less time.
6. Allow the tea to cool slightly before drinking.
7. Enjoy the tea unsweetened. If desired, add a slice of lemon without sugar for extra flavor.

NUTRITIONAL INFORMATION:

Calories: 2 | **Protein:** 0g | **Carbohydrates:** 0.5g | **Dietary Fiber:** 0g | **Sugars:** 0g | **Fat:** 0g | **Sodium:** 12mg | **Potassium:** 21mg | **Phosphorus:** 0mg

Mint Infused Water

Yield: 1 serving | **Prep time:** 5 minutes | **Cook time:** 0 minutes (plus chilling time)

INGREDIENTS:

- 1 cup of water
- 4-5 fresh mint leaves

DIRECTIONS:

1. Rinse the mint leaves under cold water.
2. Add the fresh mint leaves to a glass.
3. Fill the glass with 1 cup of water.
4. Use a spoon to gently bruise the mint leaves against the side of the glass to release their flavor.
5. Refrigerate the water for at least 1 hour, allowing the mint flavors to infuse into the water.
6. Before serving, you may remove the mint leaves or leave them in for added decoration.
7. Enjoy the mint-infused water chilled for a refreshing and hydrating drink.

NUTRITIONAL INFORMATION:

Calories: 0 | **Protein:** 0g | **Carbohydrates:** 0g | **Dietary Fiber:** 0g | **Sugars:** 0g | **Fat:** 0g | **Sodium:** 0mg | **Potassium:** 12mg (dependent on the number of mint leaves used) | **Phosphorus:** 0mg

Cucumber and Mint Juice

(No Added Sugar)

Yield: 1 serving | **Prep time:** 10 minutes | **Cook time:** 0 minutes

INGREDIENTS:

- 1 large cucumber
- A handful of fresh mint leaves
- 1/2 cup of water (optional for blending)
- Ice cubes (optional for serving)

DIRECTIONS:

1. Wash the cucumber and mint leaves thoroughly under cold water.
2. Chop the cucumber into chunks that will fit easily into your juicer or blender.
3. If using a blender, add the cucumber chunks, mint leaves, and 1/2 cup of water to the blender. Blend until smooth.
4. If using a juicer, feed the cucumber chunks and mint leaves into the juicer according to the manufacturer's instructions.
5. Once juiced or blended, strain the mixture through a fine mesh sieve or cheesecloth into a glass to remove any pulp or leaf bits, ensuring a smooth juice.
6. Add ice cubes to the glass for a desired chilled beverage.
7. Serve immediately to enjoy the refreshing and hydrating benefits of this no-added-sugar juice.

NUTRITIONAL INFORMATION:

Calories: 45 | **Protein:** 2g | **Carbohydrates:** 11g | **Dietary Fiber:** 1g | **Sugars:** 5g (naturally occurring) | **Fat:** 0.3g | **Sodium:** 6mg | **Potassium:** 442mg | **Phosphorus:** 72mg

Strawberry Basil Water

Yield: 1 serving | **Prep time:** 5 minutes | **Cook time:** 0 minutes

INGREDIENTS:

- 1 cup of water
- 3-4 fresh strawberries, sliced
- 2-3 fresh basil leaves

DIRECTIONS:

1. Combine the sliced strawberries and basil leaves in a glass or jar.
2. Fill the glass or jar with 1 cup of water.
3. Use a spoon to muddle (mash) the strawberries and basil gently leaves to release their flavors into the water.
4. Let the water infuse in the refrigerator for at least 30 minutes for the flavors to meld. Let it infuse for 1-2 hours for a more robust flavor.
5. After infusing, stir the water and strain to remove the fruit and herb pieces if desired. Alternatively, you can leave them in for a decorative look and additional flavor infusion as you drink.
6. Serve the chilled strawberry basil water for a refreshing and hydrating drink.

NUTRITIONAL INFORMATION:

Calories: 14 | **Protein:** 0.3g | **Carbohydrates:** 3.5g | **Dietary Fiber:** 1g | **Sugars:** 2.2g | **Fat:** 0.1g | **Sodium:** 3mg | **Potassium:** 85mg | **Phosphorus:** 15mg

Homemade Cranberry Juice

(Low Sugar)

Yield: 1 serving | **Prep time:** 5 minutes | **Cook time:** 20 minutes

INGREDIENTS:

- 1 cup fresh cranberries
- 2 cups water
- 1 tablespoon honey or sweetener of choice (adjust to taste)
- 1 strip of orange peel (optional for flavor)
- 1 cinnamon stick (optional for flavor)

DIRECTIONS:

1. Combine the cranberries, water, orange peel, and cinnamon stick in a medium saucepan. Bring to a boil over high heat.
2. Reduce heat to low and simmer for 15-20 minutes until the cranberries burst and the mixture slightly thickens.
3. Remove from heat and let cool slightly. Remove the orange peel and cinnamon stick.
4. Pour the mixture through a fine mesh strainer into a bowl, pressing the cranberries to extract all the juice. Discard the solids.
5. Stir in the honey or sweetener, adjusting to your preferred sweetness.
6. Chill the juice in the refrigerator until cold, or serve over ice immediately.
7. Enjoy your homemade, low-sugar cranberry juice.

NUTRITIONAL INFORMATION:

Calories: 72 | **Protein:** 0.4g | **Carbohydrates:** 19g | **Dietary Fiber:** 4.6g | **Sugars:** 12g (varies depending on the amount and type of sweetener used) | **Fat:** 0.1g | **Sodium:** 5mg | **Potassium:** 85mg | **Phosphorus:** 10mg

Chamomile Tea
(Unsweetened)

Yield: 1 serving | **Prep time:** 2 minutes | **Cook time:** 5 minutes

INGREDIENTS:

- 1 cup water
- 1 chamomile tea bag

DIRECTIONS:

1. Boil 1 cup of water in a kettle or pot.
2. Place the chamomile tea bag in a mug.
3. Once the water has reached a rolling boil, pour it over the tea bag in the mug.
4. Depending on your preferred strength, Allow the tea to steep for 3-5 minutes.
5. Remove the tea bag from the mug. For a weaker tea, steep for a shorter time.
6. Let the tea cool for a moment before drinking.
7. Enjoy the tea unsweetened, experiencing chamomile's natural, subtle sweetness and calming properties.

NUTRITIONAL INFORMATION:

Calories: 2 | **Protein:** 0g | **Carbohydrates:** 0.5g | **Dietary Fiber:** 0g | **Sugars:** 0g | **Fat:** 0g | **Sodium:** 12mg | **Potassium:** 21mg | **Phosphorus:** 0mg

Ginger Lemonade
(No Added Sugar)

Yield: 1 serving | **Prep time:** 10 minutes | **Cook time:** 0 minutes

INGREDIENTS:

- 1 cup of water
- Juice of 1/2 lemon
- 1 teaspoon fresh ginger, grated
- Ice cubes (optional)
- Fresh mint leaves for garnish (optional)

DIRECTIONS:

1. Combine the lemon juice and grated ginger in a glass with 1 cup of water. Stir well to mix.
2. Add ice cubes to the glass for a desired chilled beverage.
3. Let the mixture sit for 5 minutes to allow the ginger to infuse into the water.
4. Strain the lemonade to remove the ginger pulp, if preferred.
5. Garnish with fresh mint leaves for an extra refreshing taste.
6. Serve immediately and enjoy this revitalizing, kidney-friendly drink.

NUTRITIONAL INFORMATION:

Calories: 6 | **Protein:** 0.2g | **Carbohydrates:** 2g | **Dietary Fiber:** 0.3g | **Sugars:** 0.6g (naturally occurring from lemon) | **Fat:** 0.1g | **Sodium:** 1mg | **Potassium:** 31mg | **Phosphorus:** 4mg

CHAPTER 11

A 12-Week Meal Plan

—

Week 1

DAY	BREAKFAST	LUNCH	DINNER	DESSERT
Mon	Low-Sodium Scrambled Eggs	Grilled Chicken Salad with Low-Sodium Dressing	Grilled Lemon-Herb Chicken Breast	Vanilla Rice Pudding
Tue	Renal-Friendly Apple Cinnamon Oatmeal	Tuna Salad Sandwich on Low-Sodium Bread	Baked Cod with Parsley Pesto	Baked Cinnamon Apples
Wed	Kidney Care Blueberry Smoothie	Renal-Friendly Chicken Wrap	Low-Sodium Beef Stroganoff	Low-Potassium Berry Parfait
Thu	Low-Potassium Pancakes	Egg Salad with Low-Sodium Mayonnaise	Kidney-Friendly Turkey Meatloaf	Honey-Glazed Grilled Peaches
Fri	Egg White Omelette with Herbs	Vegetable Stir-Fry with White Rice	Lemon Pepper Baked Salmon	Angel Food Cake with Fresh Strawberries
Sat	Rice Porridge with Apples	Quinoa Salad with Lemon Vinaigrette	Quinoa Stuffed Bell Peppers	Lemon Sorbet
Sun	Low-Sodium French Toast	Baked Lemon Pepper Cod	Eggplant Parmesan with Low-Phosphorus Cheese	Blueberry Crisp with Oat Topping

Week 2

DAY	BREAKFAST	LUNCH	DINNER	DESSERT
Mon	Creamy Polenta with Fresh Berries	Quinoa Salad with Lemon Vinaigrette	Eggplant Parmesan with Low-Phosphorus Cheese	Baked Custard (Low Phosphorus)
Tue	Baked Sweet Potato with Cinnamon	Vegetable Stir-Fry with White Rice	Garlic Shrimp with Zucchini Noodles	Low-Potassium Berry Parfait
Wed	Renal Diet Veggie Frittata	Lentil Soup (Low Potassium Recipe)	Quinoa Stuffed Bell Peppers	Lemon Sorbet
Thu	Kidney-Friendly Smoothie Bowl	Baked Lemon Pepper Cod	Sautéed Lemon Garlic Scallops	Honey-Glazed Grilled Peaches
Fri	Oatmeal with Sliced Peaches	Tuna Salad Sandwich on Low-Sodium Bread	Pan-Seared Pork Chops with Apples	Angel Food Cake with Fresh Strawberries
Sat	Low-Potassium Bagel with Cream Cheese	Greek Salad with Feta (Low Sodium)	Low-Sodium Beef Stroganoff	Coconut Rice Pudding
Sun	Chia Seed Pudding with Berries	Turkey and Avocado Sandwich on Low-Sodium Bread	Baked Chicken with Thyme and Vegetables	Almond Flour Shortbread Cookies

Week 3

DAY	BREAKFAST	LUNCH	DINNER	DESSERT
Mon	Renal-Friendly Apple Cinnamon Oatmeal	Grilled Chicken Salad with Low-Sodium Dressing	Quinoa Stuffed Bell Peppers	Vanilla Rice Pudding
Tue	Low-Potassium Bagel with Cream Cheese	Baked Lemon Pepper Cod	Oven-Baked Tilapia with Fresh Herbs	Baked Cinnamon Apples
Wed	Kidney-Friendly Banana Bread	Vegetable Stir-Fry with White Rice	Lemon Pepper Baked Salmon	Low-Potassium Berry Parfait
Thu	Berry and Almond Yogurt Parfait	Tuna Salad Sandwich on Low-Sodium Bread	Eggplant Parmesan with Low-Phosphorus Cheese	Honey-Glazed Grilled Peaches
Fri	Savory Oatmeal with Egg Whites	Cauliflower Rice and Vegetable Medley	Asian-Style Tofu Stir-Fry with Vegetables	Angel Food Cake with Fresh Strawberries
Sat	Baked Peach Oatmeal	Quinoa Salad with Lemon Vinaigrette	Garlic Shrimp with Zucchini Noodles	Lemon Sorbet
Sun	Kidney Care Fruit Salad	Lentil Soup (Low Potassium Recipe)	Low-Sodium Chicken Tikka Masala	Coconut Rice Pudding

Week 4

DAY	BREAKFAST	LUNCH	DINNER	DESSERT
Mon	Egg White and Tomato Scramble	Grilled Shrimp with Garlic and Herbs	Oven-Baked Tilapia with Fresh Herbs	Vanilla Rice Pudding
Tue	Creamy Rice Cereal with Apples	Beef Stir-Fry with Low-Sodium Soy Sauce	Quinoa Salad with Roasted Vegetables	Baked Cinnamon Apples
Wed	Kidney Care Fruit Salad	Vegetable Sushi Rolls with Low-Sodium Soy Sauce	Grilled Lemon-Herb Chicken Breast	Low-Potassium Berry Parfait
Thu	Low-Phosphorus Cheese Omelette	Ratatouille with Eggplant and Zucchini	Garlic Shrimp with Zucchini Noodles	Honey-Glazed Grilled Peaches
Fri	Banana and Blueberry Pancakes	Couscous Salad with Roasted Vegetables	Asian-Style Tofu Stir-Fry with Vegetables	Angel Food Cake with Fresh Strawberries
Sat	Baked Sweet Potato with Cinnamon	Egg Salad with Low-Sodium Mayonnaise	Low-Sodium Beef Stroganoff	Lemon Sorbet
Sun	Quinoa Porridge with Mixed Berries	Tuna Salad Sandwich on Low-Sodium Bread	Eggplant Parmesan with Low-Phosphorus Cheese	Coconut Rice Pudding

Week 5

DAY	BREAKFAST	LUNCH	DINNER	DESSERT
Mon	Savory Oatmeal with Egg Whites	Vegetable Stir-Fry with White Rice	Oven-Baked Sweet Potato with Cinnamon (Small Portion)	Baked Custard (Low Phosphorus)
Tue	Baked Peach Oatmeal	Lentil Soup (Low Potassium Recipe)	Quinoa Stuffed Bell Peppers	Lemon Ricotta Cheesecake (Low-Phosphorus)
Wed	Renal Diet Veggie Frittata	Grilled Shrimp with Garlic and Herbs	Lemon Pepper Baked Salmon	Low-Phosphorus Chocolate Mousse
Thu	Rice Porridge with Apples	Couscous Salad with Roasted Vegetables	Eggplant Parmesan with Low-Phosphorus Cheese	Poached Pears in White Wine
Fri	Kidney Care Blueberry Smoothie	Baked Lemon Pepper Cod	Garlic Shrimp with Zucchini Noodles	Strawberry Gelatin with Whipped Topping
Sat	Creamy Polenta with Fresh Berries	Ratatouille with Eggplant and Zucchini	Grilled Lemon-Herb Chicken Breast	Honey-Glazed Grilled Peaches
Sun	Low-Potassium Bagel with Cream Cheese	Tuna Salad Sandwich on Low-Sodium Bread	Low-Sodium Beef Stroganoff	Vanilla Rice Pudding

Week 6

DAY	BREAKFAST	LUNCH	DINNER	DESSERT
Mon	Creamy Polenta with Fresh Berries	Grilled Chicken Salad with Low-Sodium Dressing	Baked Cod with Parsley Pesto	Coconut Rice Pudding
Tue	Low-Potassium Potato Pancakes	Vegetable Stir-Fry with White Rice	Garlic Shrimp with Zucchini Noodles	Baked Pears with Honey and Cinnamon
Wed	Baked Sweet Potato with Cinnamon	Tuna Salad Sandwich on Low-Sodium Bread	Quinoa Stuffed Bell Peppers	Lemon Sorbet
Thu	Kidney-Friendly Granola with Almond Milk	Couscous Salad with Roasted Vegetables	Oven-Baked Tilapia with Fresh Herbs	Almond Flour Shortbread Cookies
Fri	Low-Sodium Vegetable Quiche	Lentil Soup (Low Potassium Recipe)	Lemon Pepper Baked Salmon	Vanilla Rice Pudding
Sat	Pearled Barley with Cinnamon and Nutmeg	Baked Lemon Pepper Cod	Grilled Lemon-Herb Chicken Breast	Low-Potassium Berry Parfait
Sun	Renal Diet Veggie Frittata	Ratatouille with Eggplant and Zucchini	Low-Sodium Beef Stroganoff	Honey-Glazed Grilled Peaches

Week 7

DAY	BREAKFAST	LUNCH	DINNER	DESSERT
Mon	Low-Sodium Scrambled Eggs	Quinoa Salad with Lemon Vinaigrette	Grilled Lemon-Herb Chicken Breast	Vanilla Rice Pudding
Tue	Renal-Friendly Apple Cinnamon Oatmeal	Vegetable Stir-Fry with White Rice	Oven-Baked Tilapia with Fresh Herbs	Baked Cinnamon Apples
Wed	Kidney Care Blueberry Smoothie	Baked Lemon Pepper Cod	Quinoa Stuffed Bell Peppers	Low-Potassium Berry Parfait
Thu	Low-Potassium Pancakes	Grilled Chicken Salad with Low-Sodium Dressing	Garlic Shrimp with Zucchini Noodles	Honey-Glazed Grilled Peaches
Fri	Creamy Polenta with Fresh Berries	Lentil Soup (Low Potassium Recipe)	Eggplant Parmesan with Low-Phosphorus Cheese	Angel Food Cake with Fresh Strawberries
Sat	Baked Peach Oatmeal	Tuna Salad Sandwich on Low-Sodium Bread	Low-Sodium Beef Stroganoff	Lemon Sorbet
Sun	Berry and Almond Yogurt Parfait	Cauliflower Rice and Vegetable Medley	Lemon Pepper Baked Salmon	Coconut Rice Pudding

Week 8

DAY	BREAKFAST	LUNCH	DINNER	DESSERT
Mon	Low-Sodium Scrambled Eggs	Tuna Salad Sandwich on Low-Sodium Bread	Oven-Baked Tilapia with Fresh Herbs	Poached Pears in White Wine
Tue	Renal Diet Veggie Frittata	Beef Stew with Low-Potassium Vegetables	Eggplant Parmesan with Low-Phosphorus Cheese	Coconut Rice Pudding
Wed	Rice Porridge with Apples	Quinoa Salad with Lemon Vinaigrette	Garlic Shrimp with Zucchini Noodles	Apple Crumble with Oat Topping
Thu	Berry and Almond Yogurt Parfait	Vegetable Stir-Fry with White Rice	Quinoa Stuffed Bell Peppers	Grilled Banana with Honey Glaze
Fri	Baked Apples with Cinnamon	Lentil Soup (Low Potassium Recipe)	Lemon Pepper Baked Salmon	Strawberry Gelatin with Whipped Topping
Sat	Pineapple Rice Pudding	Couscous Salad with Roasted Vegetables	Stuffed Peppers with Quinoa and Vegetables	Low-Sodium Apple Pie
Sun	Kidney-Friendly Smoothie Bowl	Egg White Scramble with Asparagus	Grilled Portobello Mushrooms	Chia Seed Pudding with Almond Milk

Week 9

DAY	BREAKFAST	LUNCH	DINNER	DESSERT
Mon	Creamy Rice Cereal with Apples	Chicken Caesar Salad (No Anchovies)	Sautéed Lemon Garlic Scallops	Almond Flour Shortbread Cookies
Tue	Savory Oatmeal with Egg Whites	Ratatouille with Eggplant and Zucchini	Low-Sodium Chicken Tikka Masala	Watermelon and Feta Salad
Wed	Pearled Barley with Cinnamon and Nutmeg	Vegetable and Barley Stew	Grilled Polenta with Roasted Vegetables	Low-Sodium Apple Pie
Thu	Low-Phosphorus Cheese Omelette	Beef Stir-Fry with Low-Sodium Soy Sauce	Kidney-Friendly Pasta Primavera	Peach Cobbler with Low-Phosphorus Biscuit Topping
Fri	Egg White and Tomato Scramble	Vegetable Sushi Rolls with Low-Sodium Soy Sauce	Oven-Baked Sweet Potato with Cinnamon (Small Portion)	Mixed Berry Salad with Mint
Sat	Breakfast Rice Bowl with Mixed Veggies	Tofu and Broccoli Stir-Fry	Herbed Chicken and Vegetable Skillet	Baked Pears with Honey and Cinnamon
Sun	Baked Peach Oatmeal	Greek Salad with Feta (Low Sodium)	Fish Tacos with Cabbage Slaw	Berry and Yogurt Smoothie

Week 10

DAY	BREAKFAST	LUNCH	DINNER	DESSERT
Mon	Rice Cake with Almond Butter	Rice and Beans with Low-Sodium Seasoning	Lemon Pepper Baked Salmon	Poached Pears in White Wine
Tue	Carrot and Zucchini Muffins (low-potassium)	Greek Salad with Feta (Low Sodium)	Baked Haddock with Parsley Sauce	Grilled Banana with Honey Glaze
Wed	Baked Sweet Potato with Cinnamon	Vegetable Stir-Fry with White Rice	Low-Sodium Chicken Noodle Soup	Lemon Sorbet
Thu	Tofu Scramble with Vegetables	Broiled White Fish with Herbs	Stir-Fried Tofu with Mixed Vegetables	Strawberry Gelatin with Whipped Topping
Fri	Low-Potassium Potato Pancakes	Baked Sweet Potato (small portion) with Cinnamon	Quinoa Salad with Roasted Vegetables	Low-Phosphorus Chocolate Mousse
Sat	Renal-Friendly Cranberry Muffins	Stuffed Bell Peppers (Low Potassium)	Low-Sodium Beef Stroganoff	Baked Custard (Low Phosphorus)
Sun	Quinoa Porridge with Mixed Berries	Egg White Scramble with Asparagus	Grilled Polenta with Roasted Vegetables	Coconut Rice Pudding

Week 11

DAY	BREAKFAST	LUNCH	DINNER	DESSERT
Mon	Creamy Polenta with Fresh Berries	Chicken and Rice Casserole (Low Sodium)	Grilled Lemon-Herb Chicken Breast	Mixed Berry Salad with Mint
Tue	Savory Oatmeal with Egg Whites	Spinach and Mushroom Quiche (Egg Whites)	Garlic Shrimp with Zucchini Noodles	Blueberry Crisp with Oat Topping
Wed	Kidney-Friendly Banana Bread	Baked Sweet Potato (small portion) with Cinnamon	One-Pan Balsamic Chicken and Veggies	Poached Pears in White Wine
Thu	Pineapple Rice Pudding (with low-potassium pineapples)	Tofu and Broccoli Stir-Fry	Baked Haddock with Parsley Sauce	Lemon Ricotta Cheesecake (Low-Phosphorus)
Fri	Low-Phosphorus Muesli	Beef Stir-Fry with Low-Sodium Soy Sauce	Stir-Fried Tofu with Mixed Vegetables	Low-Phosphorus Chocolate Mousse
Sat	Renal Diet Veggie Frittata	Vegetarian Chili with Kidney Beans	Low-Sodium Beef Stroganoff	Coconut Rice Pudding
Sun	Quinoa Porridge with Mixed Berries	Vegetable Sushi Rolls with Low-Sodium Soy Sauce	Quinoa Salad with Roasted Vegetables	Angel Food Cake with Fresh Strawberries

Week 12

DAY	BREAKFAST	LUNCH	DINNER	DESSERT
Mon	Low-Sodium Scrambled Eggs	Grilled Chicken Salad with Low-Sodium Dressing	Grilled Lemon-Herb Chicken Breast	Vanilla Rice Pudding
Tue	Renal-Friendly Apple Cinnamon Oatmeal	Tuna Salad Sandwich on Low-Sodium Bread	Baked Cod with Parsley Pesto	Baked Cinnamon Apples
Wed	Kidney Care Blueberry Smoothie	Renal-Friendly Chicken Wrap	Low-Sodium Beef Stroganoff	Low-Potassium Berry Parfait
Thu	Low-Potassium Pancakes	Egg Salad with Low-Sodium Mayonnaise	Kidney-Friendly Turkey Meatloaf	Honey-Glazed Grilled Peaches
Fri	Egg White Omelette with Herbs	Vegetable Stir-Fry with White Rice	Lemon Pepper Baked Salmon	Angel Food Cake with Fresh Strawberries
Sat	Rice Porridge with Apples	Low-Potassium Tomato Soup	Quinoa Stuffed Bell Peppers	Lemon Sorbet
Sun	Berry and Almond Yogurt Parfait	Quinoa Salad with Lemon Vinaigrette	Eggplant Parmesan with Low-Phosphorus Cheese	Blueberry Crisp with Oat Topping

CHAPTER 12 **(BONUS CHAPTER)**

A Key to Managing Kidney Disease

Living with kidney disease presents not just physical challenges but also profound impacts on mental health. While dietary adjustments are often the focus of managing kidney disease, addressing psychological well-being is equally crucial. This article explores the significance of nurturing mental health and offers strategies to manage stress, enhancing the quality of life for those affected by kidney disease.

THE MENTAL HEALTH-KIDNEY DISEASE CONNECTION

Kidney disease, with its long-term implications and treatment demands, can be a source of significant stress, anxiety, and depression for patients. The uncertainties surrounding disease progression, lifestyle adjustments, and potential dialysis can take a toll on one's mental health. Recognizing and addressing these psychological aspects is vital in the holistic management of kidney disease.

STRATEGIES FOR ENHANCING MENTAL WELL-BEING

- **Professional Support:** Seeking the guidance of mental health professionals can provide coping mechanisms to deal with stress, anxiety, and depression. Therapies such as Cognitive Behavioral Therapy (CBT) have been shown to be effective in managing chronic illness-related stress.

- **Peer Support Groups:** Connecting with others who are going through similar experiences can provide comfort and reduce feelings of isolation. Peer support groups offer a platform for sharing tips, experiences, and emotional support.

- **Mindfulness and Relaxation Techniques:** Practices such as meditation, yoga, and deep-breathing exercises can reduce stress levels and improve mental health. These techniques help in focusing on the present moment and reducing negative thoughts related to the future.

- **Physical Activity:** Regular, moderate exercise suitable for one's physical condition can boost mood by releasing endorphins, known as the body's natural stress reliever. Activities should be chosen in consultation with healthcare providers to ensure they are safe and appropriate.

- **Hobbies and Interests:** Engaging in hobbies and interests can offer a sense of normalcy and joy, diverting attention from the disease. Whether it's reading, gardening, or any other leisure activity, spending time on what you love can have therapeutic effects.

CONCLUSION

Managing kidney disease extends beyond physical care to encompass mental health. By adopting a comprehensive approach that includes support for psychological well-being, individuals can face the challenges of kidney disease with resilience and improved quality of life. Remember, taking care of your mind is just as important as taking care of your body, especially when navigating the complexities of chronic illness.

Measure conversion chart

CUP	TABLESPOONS (tbsp)	TEASPOONS (tsp)	FLUID OUNCES (oz)	MILLILITERS (ml)
1	16	48	8	237
3/4	12	36	6	177
2/3	10 + 2 tsp	32	5 1/3	158
1/2	8	24	4	118
1/3	5 + 1 tsp	16	2 2/3	79
1/4	4	12	2	59
1/6	2 + 2 tsp	8	1 1/3	40
1/8	2	6	1	30
1/16	1	3	1/2	15

Renal diet food list

CHECK LABEL FOR: **(S) SODIUM** ● | **(PO) POTASSIUM** ▲ | **(PH) PHOSPHORUS** ■

25 Best Foods To Eat ★

- Arugula (1 cup, raw)
  S:6mg, PO:74mg, PH:10mg
- Bell Peppers (1, small)
  S:3mg, PO:156mg, PH:19mg
- Cabbage (1 cup)
  S:13mg, PO:119mg, PH:18mg
- Cauliflower (1 cup)
  S:19mg, PO:176mg, PH:40mg
- Garlic (3 cloves)
  S:1.5mg, PO:36mg, PH:14mg
- Onions (1, small)
  S:3mg, PO:102mg, PH:20mg
- Radishes (½ cup)
  S:23mg, PO:135mg, PH:12mg
- Shiitake Mushroom (1 c.)
  S:6mg, PO:170mg, PH:42mg
- Turnips (½ cup)
  S:13mg, PO:138mg, PH:20mg
- Parsley (1 tablespoon)
  S:2mg, PO:21mg, PH:2.2mg
- Apples (1, medium)
  S:0mg, PO:158mg, PH:10mg
- Blueberries (1 cup)
  S:1.5mg, PO:114mg, PH:18mg
- Cherries (½ cup)
  S:0mg, PO:160mg, PH:15mg
- Cranberries (1 cup)
  S:2mg, PO:80mg, PH:11mg
- Pineapple (1 cup)
  S:2mg, PO:180mg, PH:20mg
- Raspberries (½ cup)
  S:0mg, PO:93mg, PH:7mg
- Red Grapes (1 cup)
  S:3mg, PO:288mg, PH:30mg
- Strawberries (½ cup)
  S:1mg, PO:120mg, PH:13mg
- Buckwheat (½ cup)
  S:3.5mg, PO:74mg, PH:59mg
- Bulgur (½ cup)
  S:4.5mg, PO:62mg, PH:36mg
- Egg Whites (2 large)
  S:110mg, PO:108mg, PH:10mg
- Sea Bass (3 oz.)
  S:74mg, PO:279mg, PH:211mg
- Skinless Chicken (3 oz.)
  S:63mg, PO:216mg, PH:192mg
- Macadamia Nuts (1 oz.)
  S:1.4mg, PO:103mg, PH:53mg
- Olive Oil (1 tablespoon)
  S:0.3mg, PO:0.1mg, PH:0mg

Vegetables

- Alfalfa
- Asparagus
- Arugula ★
- Bamboo Shoots
- Bean Sprouts
- Bell Pepper ★
- Broccoli
- Cabbage ★
- Carrots
- Cauliflower ★
- Celery
- Chili Peppers
- Chives
- Cilantro
- Collard Greens
- Corn
- Cucumbers
- Eggplant
- Endive
- Escarole
- Green Beans
- Garlic ★
- Hominy
- Kale
- Leeks
- Lettuce
- Mushrooms ★
- Okra
- Onions ★
- Parsley ★
- Peapods/Peas
- Pimientos
- Radishes ★
- Rhubarb
- Shallots
- Spaghetti squash
- Spinach
- Sugar Snap Peas
- Summer Squash
- Turnips ★
- Turnip Greens
- Water Chestnuts (Canned)
- Watercress
- Wax Beans
- Yellow Beans
- Zucchini

Fruit

- Apples ★
- Applesauce
- Blackberries
- Blueberries ★
- Boysenberries
- Cherries ★
- Clementine
- Cranberries ★
- Fruit Cocktail
- Gooseberries
- Grapes
- Grapefruit
- Honeydew Melon
- Lemons
- Limes
- Mandarin Oranges
- Mulberries
- Peaches
- Pears
- Pineapple ★
- Plums
- Red Grapes ★
- Rhubarb
- Raspberries ★
- Strawberries ★
- Tangerines
- Watermelon

Animal Protein

- Beef (Lean Cuts)
- Chicken (Skinless) ■ ★
- Duck (Skinless) ■
- Eggs (Egg Whites) ★
- Fish
- Lamb
- Pork (Lean Cuts)
- Salmon ■
- Sea Bass ■ ★
- Shellfish ■
- Tuna (Canned, in water) ■
- Turkey (Skinless) ■
- Wild Game

Plant Protein

- Beans (Dried) ▲ ■
- Beans (Canned) ● ▲ ■
- Chickpeas ●
- Lentils ▲ ■
- Nuts (Unsalted) ● ▲ ★
- Nut Butter
- Seeds (Unsalted) ▲ ■
- Seitan
- Tempeh
- Tofu ● ▲

Dairy

- Butter (Unsalted)
- Cheese (Low Sodium)
- Cottage Cheese ● ▲
- Milk (Plant Based) ▲ ■
- Milk, Cows (1% or Skim) ▲
- Yogurt ▲ ■

Grains/Cereals

- Buckwheat ★
- Bulgur ★
- Bread ■
- Pasta
- Pretzels (Unsalted) ●
- Cereal (Unsweetened)
- Crackers (Low Sodium) ●
- Oatmeal
- Popcorn Kernals
- Quinoa ● ■
- Rice

Treats & Snacks

- Cake (Angel or Yellow)
- Fruit Snacks
- Gumdrops
- Hard Candy
- Ice Cream ● ■
- Jelly Beans
- Marshmallows
- Pie (Low-Potassium Fruit)
- Sorbet

Spices/Flavoring

- Allspice
- Canola Oil
- Chili Powder
- Cinnamon
- Coconut Aminos
- Cumin
- Curry
- Extracts (Almond, Vanilla)
- Garlic Powder
- Herbs (Dried or Fresh)
- Honey
- Hummus ●
- Jelly/Jam
- Nutmeg
- Nutritional Yeast
- Olive Oil ★
- Onion Powder
- Paprika
- Salsa ● ▲
- Sauces (Low Sodium) (BBQ, Chili, Hot, etc.) ● ▲
- Vinegar (Balsamic, Red Wine, Apple Cider, etc.)
- Zest (Lemon, Lime)

Beverages

- Coffee
- Fruit Juices (Sugar-Free)
- Seltzer Water ■
- Soda (Clear, Diet)
- Tea (Unsweetened)

Made in the USA
Monee, IL
20 June 2024